Lyme Whisperer

Lyme Whisperer

The Secret's Out

We're not crazy! And we're not alone!

Joy Pelletier Devins

www.lymewhisperer.com
https://www.facebook.com/LymeWhisperer

Library of Congress Control Number:		2014920001
ISBN:	Hardcover	978-1-5035-1413-3
	Softcover	978-1-5035-1414-0
	eBook	978-1-5035-1412-6

Rev. date: 11/12/2014

To order additional copies of this book, contact:
Xlibris
1-888-795-4274
www.Xlibris.com
Orders@Xlibris.com
633601

Contents

Foreword

Nathan Morris, MD

What an honor to precede such a wonderful and necessary book! This book is valuable in so many ways. It's important for patients who have Lyme and the need for community, as well as for physicians who have the need to better understand the daily travails of our patients.

Most patients who have Lyme disease don't have the energy or the words to describe what they go through in their process of healing. Let this book act as that catharsis. We are fortunate, indeed, to take a peek into Joy's experience and identify with her wonderful anger, frustrations, and struggles along the way, written in a witty and empathetic fashion.

People who read this book will find insight and hope, and most importantly, they will learn that they and their families are not alone. It will validate their hopes, fears, and pain, leaving them with a sense of community and camaraderie. With this will also come a deeper understanding and appreciation for the uniqueness of your own healing path. As I have found in my practice, if you have met one Lyme patient, you have not met them all. Each individual journey is unique and distinctive.

I met Joy on my own journey into Lyme, purely by serendipity. I was working on my own salvation from standardized medicine. I had turned to functional medicine instead, a model of practicing medicine that treats the whole person and addresses the underlying causes of the disease while building a therapeutic patient-and-practitioner partnership. While on this journey into functional medicine, our paths, fortunately, crossed. When I am with Joy, I am amazed at her spirit and the humor that defines her. It is not this disease called Lyme that defines her. I think this is so important. You are a patient who has Lyme, not a Lyme patient. Joy personifies this.

I had been having a fine time treating patients through the functional medicine paradigm, until the really complex cases kept leading to Lyme. I realized that a large number of patients were walking through my door after seeing countless professionals and that they still had no answers. I started to see the light and *panicked!* Suddenly my journey out of traditional medicine and into functional medicine had led me kicking and screaming straight into the world of Lyme. Identifying Lyme is not easy, but finding someone to treat it, or even to *help me* treat it, was almost impossible.

Though treating Lyme downright scares me at times, I know I have to face what is in front of me at the moment. What is in front of me is a whole mess of people that need care, compassion, and above all, hope. I have noticed this: The people who do the best are the ones who don't let this disease define them. They fight it and choose to find happiness despite it.

I make this bargain with my patients: I will never stop learning if you never give up. My patients are my greatest inspiration and my greatest teachers. I feel fortunate indeed and there is so much to learn every day.

This book is a great tool in the fight to keep your head—and spirits—above the water. May its boisterous vigor bring you some laughs and shine a light for you in sometimes dark places.

Read more about Dr. Nathan in chapter 5's "The Coow Woow Interview with Dr. Nathan."

Preface

Psssst. It's me. The Lyme Whisperer. I wrote this book to share a secret. Come closer. Don't worry, I don't bite. Ticks bite. So here goes. *Lyme sufferers are not crazy*. Their bizarre symptoms are not all in their head. And chronic Lyme disease is real. Now, whatever you do, don't *not* go around telling everyone that you know.

I am a thirty-nine-year-old mom, wife, vice president, runner, community volunteer, and blogger.

I was diagnosed with Lyme disease in November of 2010 after two years of symptoms. Until then, I felt crazy and alone. No one understood my terror and frustration. And it seemed that no one *really* wanted to help. I felt abandoned by a medical community that, purposely or not, turned their backs on me.

My muscles twitched constantly, from my eyelids to my ankles. Buzzing sensations made it feel like cell phones were vibrating in my legs and feet. I always had pins and needles in my extremities. Electric shocks surged through my forearms like I was short-circuiting. Sometimes it seemed like someone was tightening a belt around my abdomen. My big toe felt like it was crossed over the second toe even though it wasn't. I was dizzy, and sometimes, the whole room would suddenly tilt. My ears were ringing, and I had ear and jaw pain. I had stabbing pains in the back of my head and behind my right eye. I also had lots of floaters and saw double images. At times, it felt like ants were crawling under my skin. At other times, it felt like warm water was running down my legs. My psoriasis flared like it had never flared before. Impossibly heavy menstrual cycles became impossibly heavier. I was forgetful and absentminded. I would walk into a room and forget why. I would get lost driving in my neighborhood or on the way to work. I experienced crushing fatigue. My back was in agonizing pain. My bladder was inflamed, and I feared the powerful, painful bladder spasms. I went from never having sinus infections to always having sinus infections. Panic attacks consumed me.

I visited specialist after specialist, chasing my symptoms, including a urologist, optometrist, Ob-gyn, chiropractor, dermatologist, and neurologist. I ended up in the ER twice. I had MRIs, CAT scans, chest x-rays, EKGs, ultrasounds, biopsies, blood tests, and more blood tests. Celiac disease, diabetes, multiple sclerosis, a brain tumor, and uterine cancer were among the things that were ruled out. "Nothing" was wrong was all I heard. The neurologist told me I was just a stressed-out working mom and to go home and try to relax.

Then, I landed in the office of my Lyme-literate naturopathic doctor, though I didn't know she was Lyme literate at the time. I told her that I came to her because I was falling apart. And that it seemed like I was constantly trying to put out new fires as ailments kept mysteriously popping up. I explained that I had already spent two years going to other doctors. And that, meanwhile, I had lost twenty pounds, feared my kids were going to lose their mother, and was considering a medical leave of absence from work. Before she started trying to remedy all the different things that were wrong with me, she did *two* things. First, she continued to listen. Second, she tested me for Lyme disease.

It *was* Lyme disease. She was right. I was too physically and emotionally drained to dwell on how so many doctors had failed me until then. I put all my energy into following her ever-evolving treatment protocols of antibiotics, herbs, tinctures, probiotics, and more. She dared to care for me, and I love her for it.

I also developed my *own* form of therapy shortly thereafter. In my head, I would talk or "whisper" to Borrelia, the spiral-shaped bacteria that cause Lyme disease. I awoke one morning and angrily scolded her (Borrelia). I insisted that she was *not* going to keep me from my son's baseball game, or anything else, despite her biting into my spinal cord like a Doberman with a rope toy. I defied Borrelia that morning by verbally taking the upper hand, and I've been whispering to her ever since.

That is how the Lyme Whisperer came to be. I began to chronicle my thoughts and conversations aimed at Borrelia as I pushed forward in my journey. My blog, LymeWhisperer.com, was created as a result. This book is based on my blog.

The aim of this book is to raise hope and awareness surrounding Lyme disease. Lyme sufferers will recognize themselves and feel validated, helping to end ongoing self-doubt. Others who have experienced mysterious symptoms without answers may relate and finally have hope for a proper diagnosis. Friends and family can finally peek into the confused and anguished mind of their loved one. The medical community can learn from a silently suffering patient's point of view and maybe even learn to recognize symptoms earlier. Secretly curious legislators will realize more must be done and faster to stop the suffering in their communities.

The cruel reality of Lyme is that the disease is only half the battle. I came across a quote from Kenneth Liegner, MD, that reads, "In the fullness of time, the mainstream handling of Chronic Lyme disease will be viewed as one of the most shameful episodes in the history of medicine because elements of academic medicine, elements of government and virtually the entire insurance industry have colluded to deny a disease."

The beauty of the very vocal Lyme community is that we ultimately refuse to be denied or ignored. We will be heard, one whisper at a time. So pass the megaphone. I'm ready to share my "secrets" in the name of Lyme awareness. Because in the end, I do believe that our voices will be heard.

Acknowledgments

I would like to thank my Lyme-literate naturopathic doctor, Dr. Julia Greenspan, for her endless courage, determination, and spunk. It takes a special person to outsmart a spirochete. And a special doctor to dare enough to do it.

Thank you to my unofficial local Lyme disease support group. We call ourselves Lyme with the Wind . . . or was it Gone with the Lyme? Kelly, Pamela, Tom, Beth, Paul, Megan, Donna, Becky, Kate, David, Lynda, Jeff—we are stronger for having walked this journey together. Love you, guys—tears, laughter, spinning rooms, unplugged fans, dimmed lights, muted phones, and all.

Thank you to my whisperers for your infinite support. These are the beautiful souls who have embraced LymeWhisperer.com and Lyme Whisperer on Facebook where we have built a safe place to share hope and humor. You are all an inspiration.

Thank you, Dr. Mark Swanson, ND, Dr. Nathan Morris, MD, and Dr. Kelly Heim, PhD, for participating in some twisted-humor interviews with the Lyme Whisperer, all in the spirit of raising awareness.

Katina Makris, thank you for unlocking something in me with your book, which freed me to finally write the last chapter of my own. Your strength and intuition are a force of nature.

Charles Balducci and John Donnally of the Tick-Borne Disease Alliance, it's an honor and privilege to have met you both during this ney. Thank you for your selfless time in speaking with me. And above all, thank you for what you do at the TBDA.

Thank you to my mum, Betty Pelletier, who was the content editor for my book. She was also my high school creative writing teacher and has encouraged and nurtured my creativity always. Carpe diem, Mum. Carpe diem! Your influence and direction on this book helped me to create a work I am most proud of.

Thank you to my dad, who did *not* edit my book but *did* edit my life. Thanks, Dad, for "correcting" my weaknesses and "underlining" my strengths.

Thank you to my twin brother, Jay, my creative director behind the cover illustration of *Yardley the Trembling Tick*. Ticks are everywhere we are, including woods, lawns and yards. Jay, thanks for always being the yin to my yang. Pisces power! And thanks to friend and artistic phenom Kelly C. Heim, PhD, for creating and bringing the illustration to life.

Thank you, family, friends, neighbors, and coworkers, for caring *so* much and for being so supportive.

Lastly, thank you to Borrelia for your "inspiration." Borrelia is none other than *Borrelia burgdorferi*, the bacteria that causes Lyme disease.

Introduction

In *Lyme Whisperer: The Secret's Out*, the reader will get to overhear two years' worth of my private conversations aimed at Borrelia, the bacteria that cause Lyme disease. They will get to be a tick on the wall, so to speak. As a result, they will hear firsthand about the mental, physical, social, and political obstacles of Lyme disease.

This book is for those with Lyme disease; those who suspect they might have Lyme; supportive or skeptical family, friends, and neighbors; and anyone whose profession can help make a difference with Lyme disease, from doctors to legislators. These conversations provide an intimate look into the often silent struggles of a largely ignored and misunderstood disease.

The book is adapted from my blog, LymeWhisperer.com. It is in the format of chronological journal entries, in which I often directly address Borrelia (or B for short). Entries about aliens, Annie, Barry Manilow, Mickey Mouse, Starbucks, and DreamWorks's *Madagascar* are all in the context of Lyme disease.

The reader will find top twenty-seven and top nine lists and analogies inspired by *Snow White*, The Chronicles of Narnia, *Alice in Wonderland*, *The Avengers, Transformers, The Perfect Storm, Gone with the Wind*, Harry Potter, *World War Z, The Polar Express*, and more. The reader will discover pieces inspired by Huffington Post articles as well as by book authors, including Mark Hyman, MD, and Katina Makris, certified intuitive healer and homeopath. Other experts join in on the fun with interviews, including Nathan Morris, MD, Mark Swanson, ND, and Kelly Heim, PhD.

Though chronological, the entries in this book can be read in any order, as haphazardly as you wish. As haphazard as Lyme disease itself.

What will this book show the reader? It will show that Lyme sufferers themselves are *not* crazy and that it is *this disease* that is sheer madness. It will show the reader that the politics and controversies surrounding Lyme are just as painfully absurd. The reader will gain a better understanding of why we so fiercely need to advocate for better care and recognition.

It will show the reader that humor and gratitude can be as infectious as Borrelia herself. I try to find reasons to laugh about Lyme and reasons to be grateful, things that aren't easy to accomplish when it comes to this disease but are important for healing and recovery.

It will show the reader that with persistence and positive thinking, there *are* best-case scenarios when it comes to Lyme disease. The reader will be surprised to read "Best-Case Scenario" in the last chapter of this book as it describes what I was able to accomplish personally and professionally, even with all the ups, downs, and sideways turns that were taking place at the same time. The book ends with "Whispers of Hope," revealing hope for the future through the work and words of Katina Makris as well as Charles Balducci, cochairman of the Tick-Borne Disease Alliance.

That's right. The secret *is* out. We are not crazy, *and* we are not alone. According to the CDC (Centers for Disease Control and Prevention), there are over three hundred thousand new cases of Lyme disease annually, and only 10 percent of these are diagnosed. According to other sources, that number may be closer to one million new cases, 34–62 percent of which become chronic Lyme. The rate at which the Lyme disease epidemic is growing has surpassed the growth rate of HIV. Unreliable diagnostic tests and the medical establishments' reluctance to recognize chronic Lyme add to the list of problems.

I know firsthand how widespread this problem is. My blog followers come from forty-three countries, including the United States, Canada, France, Australia, Germany, the United Kingdom, Spain, Poland, Russia, Japan, Saudi Arabia, Egypt, China, Pakistan, and India.

The book begins after I had just completed nine months of antibiotics. I took a four-month break from antibiotics at that time, only to resume again for another four months before ending my antibiotic treatment altogether. People often ask me what my antibiotic protocol was. To be honest, I don't really know. I know that azithromycin, doxycycline, minocycline, and rifampin were some of the ones that I took, but those are the only ones I can recall by name. I was too tired and too sick to care or take note.

Dr. Steven Harris, MD, featured in the book *Insights into Lyme Disease Treatment*, by Connie Strasheim, says the people who tend to heal from Lyme disease are those who don't know how sick they are. That described me at the time. I didn't feel the need to memorize or write down my protocols. I didn't Google anything about Lyme disease. Nothing. I just pushed through. I parented, worked, exercised, and took my medications without overthinking anything. Instead, I dove into the creative outlet that would become my blog and, eventually, my book.

Nowadays, I maintain my health and progress by exercising, following a gluten-free diet, taking dietary supplements, and trying to manage stress and getting enough rest. I'm not symptom-free. But I'm free from being Borrelia's prisoner.

Chapter 1

Trash Talk with Borrelia

***

Predator versus Alien

June 10, 2012

Watched *Alien vs. Predator* on the Syfy channel last night, Borrelia. You know I never watch the Syfy channel. But as I was flipping through, I realized that the disgusting black mucus-covered alien with nasty teeth and claws is exactly how I picture you. Utterly disgusting and carnivorous. You'd have to be to gnaw through my nerves and tissues the way you have! But, hey, did that stop me in any way from catching my son's baseball play-offs today? Hell to the no, you alien.

Mind Freak

June 14, 2012

"You're the best mommy in the world, but you are very forgetful!" said my five-year-old daughter to me this morning, Borrelia. My Lyme dementia, or Lyme-mentia, is apparent even to her. Which got me to thinking about the top fifteen ways you make me a mind freak.

1. By making me stand in the shower, trying to figure out if I have already shampooed my hair or not.
2. By making me frantically search for my cell phone while *talking* on it with my friend Katrina.
3. By making me boil lettuce instead of the pasta.
4. By making me pack barbecue and peanut butter sandwiches for my kids' lunches.
5. By making me s-s-s-s-stutter and stam-stam-stammer, especially when I am tired or s-s-s-s-stressed.
6. By not making me able to spell *Borrelia* the same way twice, Borellia.
7. By making me absentmindedly put popsicles in my son's lunch box until the teacher wrote a note home saying, "Dear parent, popsicles melt."
8. By making me lose my prescriptions somewhere between the pharmacy counter, getting into the car, and pulling into the driveway. I *don't* understand where I could have put them.
9. By making me have a brain that is a password purgatory, a graveyard for all those important but forgotten passwords that I need. Facebook, Amazon, LinkedIn, Comcast, Gmail, Bank of America! *Aaaah!*
10. By making me confused by all the light switches in my house. Why do they suddenly puzzle me so? Is this the backyard switch or the garage? Kitchen or front porch? I just don't know, but I'll get it right by the fourth try.
11. By forcing me to be a voice memo vixen. I leave myself numerous voice memos every day on my iPhone. I even need to leave voice memos to remind me to check my voice memos.
12. By turning me into a graffiti artist on my own arm. I gave up using Post-its because I was always losing them. That's when I

became known around the office for writing on my hands *and* arms all the notes I needed to get me through the day—or next five minutes.

13. By making me forget to take the vitamins that are supposed to help me with my memory.

14. By having to ask my son if I have two matching earrings after I embarrassed him one day with a mismatched pair.

15. By making me a frustrated grade school mom. Bring money for field trip, bring snack, sign permission form, buy raffle tickets, send in book order, come to book fair, bring cupcakes, bring hat for hat day, bring bike for bike day, pajama day on Thursday, popcorn day Friday, bring in box tops, sign up for movie night. I can't *take* this many details, Borrelia! My brain can't take it! I can't take you!

Battle Lines Drawn

June 16, 2012

That's right, Borrelia! I woke up today with a mission. Revise and renew my battle plan. After all that I've been reading lately, I've decided I've given my body enough of a break from antibiotics and herbal tinctures, and I need to get back on track with a formidable defense strategy.

I *can* keep my defenses up against you and I must! But that's just the beginning, B. I've also decided to arm my family with some natural tick-repellent spray *and* to protect all of us with organic lawn insecticide. Are you hearing me? I'm ready to fight on several fronts here. Yeah, these are fightin' words. *T-i-c-k-tock*, Borrelia. Ticktock.

I was determined to find diatomaceous earth this morning, or DE as it's also known, but I had no luck finding it at Home Depot. DE is described as "naturally-occurring, soft, sedimentary rock with a silica-like composition." Would you like to know how it works, Borrelia? I'm going to tell you anyway. It basically causes ticks—which you use as your vehicle (more like war tank) for transmission—to die a slow, painful death of dehydration. God, I love the sound of that.

Instead, however, I did find a natural, organic EcoSmart product and am very excited about it. The EcoSmart insect killer granules will be spread over my entire lawn, and it's reassuring that it contains only eugenol, thyme oil, peanut shells, and wintergreen oil. And get this—this one works as an octopamine blocker! Yeah, baby! That's right. The essential oils in EcoSmart block the octopamine neurotransmitter in ticks. Octopamine regulates the heart rate, movements, and metabolism of ticks. That means, according to the EcoSmart website, that blocking octopamine "results in a total breakdown of the insect's central nervous system." Geez, Borrelia, sounds exactly like what you've done to me!

Anyhoo, loving my new purchase. I also picked up some body spray insect repellent at the local natural pharmacy. Again, more protection for the entire family, Borrelia. I'm not crazy about smelling so strong and citronella-y. I just prefer it to applying DEET all the time, especially when it comes to the kids. Burt's Bees body spray herbal insect repellent contains rosemary oil, peppermint oil, cedar leaf oil, clove oil, and citronella. Lawn, check! Skin, check!

Now that I've addressed external defenses against ticks, Borrelia, let's get to the internal defenses against you! Though I have tried and been pleased with Samento, as recommended by my naturopath, I think it's time I try the Samento and Banderol double whammy. In a 2010 study conducted by the Lyme Disease Research Group of the University of New Haven, Connecticut, Samento and Banderol were shown to be effective in providing immune support against you, Borrelia. In both your spirochete *and* biofilm forms—that's quite amazing. You can see an article regarding this study on the Townsend Letter website.

Samento is a liquid Cat's Claw (Uncaria tomentosa) herbal extract, while Banderol is a liquid extract of the bark of the South American Otaba tree. Used together, they are more effective than either alone, it seems. I already have the Samento, Borrelia, and I just ordered the Banderol online today. Will chat with my naturopath first before taking the combo, but I couldn't wait to get it in my (our) hands! (Someday maybe they'll be just *my* hands again!). Oh, but there's more, my "friend!"

I am also taking out my Byron White A-L Complex again and MaitakeGold 404 liquid formulas, which I still have from my last naturopath visit! For the maximum immune boost. It's boost or bust, baby! Good night, Borrelia. Sleep tight. Though not sure how well you will sleep after our little chat this evening.

Copa Cabana

June 22, 2012

Hey, Borrelia. Do the names Barry and Bradshaw mean anything to you? Well, last night they came to my mind!

The evening began with my coworkers and me sitting at the Indigo Hotel's poolside cabana in Boston's sweltering, humid one-hundred-degree heat. We sat, joking and laughing while sweat dripped down our faces. We had refreshing cocktails and refreshing conversations.

I mean, really, what better medicine is there than being distracted from your antics for a bit with sliders, tuna tartar, and great company, Borrelia?

As I noshed on the appetizers and sipped my cosmopolitan, my thoughts went to Barry Manilow and "Copacabana." I was literally *coping* in a *cabana!* I was forgetting about you for a while in what felt like the hottest spot north of Havana! It put a smile on my face, and I chuckled.

Then my blog, LymeWhisperer.com, came up in conversation. My colleagues expressed that they liked my style and the way that I chronicled life with Lyme. They said I reminded them of Carry Bradshaw, who, on the show *Sex and the City*, wrote weekly columns and provided intriguing narrative for the show. I liked that analogy. In fact, I guess I am similar to Carrie Bradshaw. In some ways. Sort of. For instance, she's a shoe lover, and I am a lover of the rationale behind Dr. Shoemaker's Lyme Protocol. (Side note: I am a fan of the *rationale* behind the protocol, which addresses susceptibility to and treatment for mold and other toxic burdens. But I am not a fan of some of the *products* in the protocol itself. I could not comply with the cholestyramine treatment. It comes in a thickly textured powder, and I couldn't choke it down, even though I felt like it was helping. Cholestyramine is a cholesterol drug but is used in the protocol to help eliminate toxins from the body.)

From bacon-wrapped scallops to thoughts of Barry Manilow and Carrie Bradshaw, I'd say it was a great night. Feeling appreciative of my coworkers and employees for keeping Borrelia at bay last night, at least mentally!

You Know You Have Lyme When . . . the only thing *not* in your laptop bag is . . . your laptop.

Chapter 2

Born to Run

***

Me, My Kid, and a 5K

June 24, 2012

Well, well, well, Borrelia! I made a commitment a month ago to get back into running. I had stopped, as you may recall, when I was at my sickest three years ago. It was too painful to run, and I was too weak. Not that I've ever stopped moving because of you, not at all. I just modified my exercise routine to include mostly walking—power walking of course. And Wii dance. And elliptical workouts. A month ago, I decided I was feeling good and up for the challenge of running again. Today marks my first 5K, and I am running it with my son.

When I awoke this morning, in usual fashion, you were a Doberman pinscher gnawing at the small of my back as if it were a rawhide bone. Mornings for me, like many Lymies, are the worst. The pain settles overnight, and in the morning, it's helloooooo, Borrelia.

I also awoke worried about how my bladder would hold up for race day. Sometimes, I wish I could wear a scarlet letter. In this case it would be an *L* on my chest to signify Lyme disease. That way I wouldn't have to explain things all the time. Like why I always need to be close to a bathroom. Oh, well, there'll be plenty of bushes and trees to hide behind on our 5K through the woods this morning.

Despite the back pain and bladder anxiety, the excitement of sticking it to you by running a 5K brought me to my feet fast. Relatively. And the fact that my son wanted to run it with me made it that much more exciting for me. While getting myself back out there was part of my motivation for running the 5K, Borrelia, there was more to it than that.

Today, Borrelia, today we ran for Rosanne. Rosanne's Rush for Research is a charitable 501(c)(3) nonprofit organization formed in the name of Rosanne Sullivan, who passed away on October 22, 2010, from triple-negative breast cancer. Triple-negative breast cancer, Borrelia.

Even you are a walk in the park when it comes to what some other people have to battle. So today, my son and I wanted to support someone else and *their* fight. We wanted to raise money for Dana-Farber cancer hospital on behalf of Rosanne so that research for triple-negative breast cancer can advance. And maybe someday someone won't lose their mom to it.

What a great day for a 5K, Borrelia! My son and I ran and walked our way through three hot miles through woodsy terrain, and his sister joined us for the victory lap around the high school track where we finished. At one point, he said, "Wow, this is harder than I thought it would be!" To which I said, "Life is going to be harder than you think it will be too. Just like Rosanne's was harder than she thought it would be." What a great feeling when we crossed that finish line! For ourselves and Rosanne and for all the women and families affected by breast cancer. I'll never forget the image of Rosanne's pink balloons floating against the brightest of blue skies that day.

Woof Woof

July 3, 2012

Come, Borrelia. Let's listen to the radio interview streaming on WBUR.

What I did know before tuning in, Borrelia, is that dogs are better protected than we are since there is a Lyme vaccine available for them. What I didn't know was how incredibly muddied the whole vaccine saga was.

"Lyme disease is the only infection I know of where we have a safe and effective vaccine, but it's not available to the public," said Dr. Allen Steere. I heard this unsettling statement as part of a special week-long "Living with Lyme" series on WBUR, Boston's National Public Radio (NPR) news station.

Dr. Allen Steere has a long history associated with Lyme. His contributions have been controversial and complex. In some aspects, his legacy is positive, including his role in uncovering and identifying the disease as a young rheumatologist in Connecticut. On the other hand, his legacy has been tarnished due to public opinion on his role in helping the Centers for Disease Control (CDC) establish the criteria for what constitutes a positive Western blot for detecting Lyme. This criteria is widely condemned by Lyme specialists and Lyme patients alike, who argue it is an unreliable, narrow, and unscientific approach. Furthermore, Dr. Steere contributed to establishing this criteria despite a potential conflict of interest as he was helping SmithKline Beecham (or SKB, now known as GlaxoSmithKline) develop the LYMErix vaccine, which was introduced in 1998.

The alleged conflict of interest had to do with Western blots and outer surface protein A, or OspA, and how vaccine development changed their course. In the case of Lyme disease, the Western blot is a test that includes Borrelia-specific proteins of varying molecular weights, from eighteen kilodaltons to ninety-three kilodaltons. The different proteins are separated by size, from highest to lowest molecular weight, on a gel medium. The serum of an individual is run against these Borrelia-specific proteins. A reaction occurs if the serum contains an antibody to any of the individual proteins, forming a band at the location of the protein. The appearance of a band or a series of bands on the gel indicates a positive result for that protein or proteins. This would mean that the body had developed antibodies to those particular proteins, which happens only when the body has been exposed to them. Therefore, exposure to Lyme disease would be suspected based on a given number of positive bands.

The Western blot criteria, developed by the CDC with Dr. Steere's consultation, did not include a key protein specific for Lyme. This protein was OspA, with a molecular weight of thirty-one kilodaltons, which would otherwise be known as band 31. The CDC contends that the Western blot criteria they developed was never intended for diagnostic purposes but rather for surveillance purposes only. That may or may not be the case, but confusion over the criteria and how to use it continued, and in many cases, it was being used as a diagnostic tool.

To include OspA, or band 31, as part of a Western blot for Lyme would seem imperative. However, some suspect it was omitted so that production of an OspA-based vaccine could be pursued, a vaccine being developed with Dr. Steere's help.

Why would an OspA-based vaccine interfere with the OspA protein being included on a Western blot? Because if OspA-vaccinated individuals were to be tested using a Western blot with OspA included, doctors would not be able to differentiate whether a positive OspA result on band 31 was due to the vaccine or to an actual Lyme infection. It was decided upon by the CDC and others with alleged financial ties to vaccine development that the Western blot would not include OspA. The application of OspA would be reserved for the vaccine instead.

I don't know what to think, Borrelia. Maybe that was the right direction. Maybe it wasn't. But sacrificing more reliable Western blot criteria for a vaccine would have been much easier to accept if the vaccine remained available. But it was only available for four years. What happened? Why and how did it disappear seemingly as fast as a doggie treat at a dog show?

In 2002, the LYMErix vaccine was voluntarily withdrawn by the manufacturer. They cited poor sales. Poor sales appeared to have been the result, in part, of media coverage on adverse reactions, particularly musculoskeletal and arthritic-type complaints from some vaccinated individuals. Class action attorneys started firing hundreds of lawsuits at SKB, like the Red Baron firing at Snoopy.

SKB maintained that arthritic conditions did not occur at a higher rate than would be expected in the general population and that adverse reactions overall did not occur at a higher rate than they would with other types of vaccines. Scientists had in fact known beforehand that a subset of patients with a particular genetic disposition would likely experience arthritis-like symptoms as a result of taking the vaccine. Warning language of this nature accompanying the vaccine may have managed expectations for those interested in taking it, but the opportunity was missed as no such warning was provided. The media had drawn attention to the issue, and the public's fear and distrust ended up sealing the fate of the vaccine. Sales plummeted, and SKB pulled the product off the market and went home with their tail between their legs.

Why wouldn't other pharmaceutical companies be deterred after all this? The fear of hundreds of class action lawsuits has been as effective as a Beware of Dog sign. No one wanted to go anywhere near it after this.

There's no denying that the vaccine had a number of shortcomings and limitations anyway. For starters, maybe an OspA-based vaccine was truly not the best direction, given the potential number of individuals who could develop Lyme arthritis from it.

Secondly, the vaccine never became an official part of childhood or adulthood vaccination schedules. Instead, it was left to doctors to determine which patients were most likely at risk, primarily based on where they lived. But what if patients who did not live in a heavily infected area visited family, attended schools, or worked in areas that were? What if communities were more at risk than they were aware of? This left doctors with vague guidelines and much confusion on who should be vaccinated.

Third, for those that were given the vaccine, the vaccine required three shots before being effective: the initial shot, a booster shot one month later, and another booster months after that. Furthermore, the vaccine was believed to be only 80 percent effective and only effective against one predominant strain of the Lyme bacteria.

Lastly, the vaccine was developed for people between the ages of fifteen to seventy years of age, leaving out a very high-risk group—young children that spend much of their time playing outdoors.

Yes, all this is unsettling to me, Borrelia. What we've heard on this radio stream demonstrates some of the earliest political influences over Lyme disease. Fortunately, newer, more advanced Western blots have been developed since the initial Western blot criteria was established. California-based reference laboratory IGeneX is a leader in this effort with their proprietary tests. The IgG and IgM Western blots developed by them are superior because they were designed to test for more than one species of Borrelia, detect various phases of Lyme, and include additional key proteins specific for Lyme, such as OspA (band 31) and OspB (band

34). However, when it comes to the vaccine, we are left scratching our heads, wondering why we are still in a situation where anyone can bring his or her dog to the vet yet can't get vaccinations for themselves or their families. Could this setback with the initial LYMErix vaccine be a setback of epic—no epidemic—proportions?

Yes, indeed it could. As Lyme has in fact grown to be what is described as the epidemic of our time. I just want to curl up in a kennel and cry, Borrelia. I'd have better protection as a canine. Maybe I'll make an appointment with the vet.

Woof woof.

Special Note:

Writing this piece made me growl. The additional research involved was more physically draining than doing the doggie paddle against a really strong current. It was more mentally draining than trying to teach an old dog new tricks while doing the doggie paddle against a really strong current. There's a labyrinth of facts, controversies, and scientific details and nuances surrounding the issues of detection and vaccination. So much so that this Lyme brain, let alone a regular brain, can't be sure that they've gotten it all right.

If you'd like to read more on these topics, please visit LymeDiseaseAssociation.org and go to "About Lyme" then "Controversy" then "Conflicts of Interest in Lyme Rprt." Lyme.org and IGeneX.com have additional information.

Dairy-Free, Symptom-Free?

July 10, 2012

Now *this* is interesting, Borrelia. My little four-week experiment. As you know, B, most with Lyme disease do need to adopt a gluten-, dairy-, and sugar-free diet. Gluten and dairy contain proteins that can be inflammatory. Since Lyme disease is already a highly inflammatory condition, diets containing gluten and dairy can make symptoms even worse.

I've also learned from my blog followers as well as Lyme friends that many of their food sensitivities did not develop until they had Lyme disease. In fact for some, food sensitivities were one of their only symptoms.

I've been gluten-free for almost four years and really find it quite easy for the most part. But never in my wildest Stonyfield Farms dreams did I ever think I would, could, or even should go dairy-free.

Yet for four weeks, I did it, Borrelia Brie Burgdorferi! Me. I actually stopped using skim milk in my granola and cut out my midmorning Chobani snack, my side of cheddar cheese for lunch . . . and afternoon snack . . . and bedtime snack. Not to mention eliminating the feta on my salads and parmesan sprinkled on soups. I practically lived on dairy, but *I did it*.

I'm so grateful for discovering how much I enjoy almond milk, coconut milk, and coconut milk yogurts. I also realized that hummus, avocado, beans, and tapenade can spice up salads, quinoa, and brown rice, as well as or better than goat cheese or feta. I'm also grateful for small improvements in my symptoms as well. The buzzing and tingling in my hands and feet seem to have calmed. Like a baby drinking warm milk. Ha! Bad time to use that analogy?

That's right, Borrelia, my hands and feet actually felt more calm and quiet and less like live wires constantly short-circuiting. The most calm they've felt since you first began drilling away at my nerves, ruining any chance for normal neurotransmission. Just maybe, maybe by taking away a source of inflammation, my nerves were finally able to start to heal.

Or maybe it's because coconut milk—my dairy milk alternative—contains omega-3, 6, and 9 essential fatty acids, nerve-nourishing fats. Whether it was the elimination of the dairy or the addition of the essential fats or both, I'm not sure, Borrelia, but I was feeling like the Non-Dairy Queen!

Then, I cheated on purpose. To see what would happen. Within a few days, it seemed that the pins and needles in my feet and the strong electrical jolts to the heel started getting more frequent. The sensation of ants crawling under my skin also returned. Maybe it's all in my head. But I know what I should do, Borrelia. Stick to limiting my dairy intake as much as possible. I'm not sure I can commit to giving up all those gorgonzola and beet or the mozzarella and heirloom tomato salads that I so love and enjoy. But I can certainly cut out the majority of dairy a majority of the time.

It's another step toward a *full* recovery, Borrelia. Aw, what's the matter? Are you *crying* over spilled milk?

Update: I did not remain dairy-free after being off dairy for over a month. As a gluten-free, busy, working, traveling, exercising mom, I just found I needed to have cheese and yogurt in my diet or go too hungry too often! I do participate, however, in periodic detox programs in which I go dairy- and caffeine-free for several weeks or a month.

The Mad Bladder

July 18, 2012

Okay, Borrelia. If anyone can be childish, it's me. But this week, this week you win. The minute I believe I'm 90 percent recovered, you have one of your childish tantrums. Like the tantrum in my bladder, making me the Mad Bladder *all over again*. Thanks, Borrelia in Wonderland, thanks.

I'm going to stick with this theme of childish behavior for a minute. Because I think I know what's going on. I know your little Red Rover, Red Rover games you play inside of me. I can visualize you and your coinfection friends, attaching and linking to one another. And in doing so, creating a barrier! A biofilm barrier. Hmmm. Biofilm is a biobitch. Who is it in there playing with you? *Bartonella?* Yes, I can picture the two of you creating biofilm, an impenetrable protective barrier that allows you to hide from antibiotics and other treatments. And in the process, you create hybrid organisms not responsive to treatment. Is that why I continue to be the Mad Bladder? And InflameBrain? Is it the result of these, your childish biofilm games? It makes full recovery almost impossible.

Well, I've got my new playbook, Borrelia. It's called *Insights into Lyme Disease Treatment*, by Connie Strasheim, author and fellow Lyme disease sufferer. Each chapter of her new book is written by a Lyme-literate physician, sharing their experiences, approaches, challenges, and successes in treating Lyme. I'm on chapter 3, Borrelia, and getting some great tips. Maybe I'm going to throw some enzymes at you, like nattokinase supplements. Or maybe lysozyme. Or both. To eat away at the biofilm. To end Red Rover, Red Rover once and for all.

You know, B, a few things I read really struck me. For instance, in chapter 1 by Steven Harris, MD, he says the people who tend to heal from Lyme disease are those who don't know how sick they are. I would say that fits me. I don't remember if I tested positive for coinfections, and I don't want to know or ask. I don't want to know my CD57 count. CD57 refers to a subset of white blood cells that are typically depressed in chronic Lyme and may (or may not) increase with treatment. I've avoided going back to the doctor for as long as I can. I've ignored follow-up tests (not necessarily a good thing). I do want to do what Dr. Harris says his most successful patients have done—just get out there and do things, live life, and function despite the adversity.

Dr. Harris wrote something else very powerful. For the first time, I felt someone actually understood the isolation and self-doubt you have made me feel, Borrelia. Dr. Harris writes, "People with Lyme disease are generally really sick, and have been this way for a long time, but their families, doctors or friends sometimes don't believe that they are unwell . . . As a result, they feel isolated as if they have been living in a twilight zone, or are going crazy. So they develop a mistrust of others, and even of themselves, and they start questioning whether they are legitimately sick. The second-guessing and this burden of guilt that people develop from being so pushed aside, is the number one most difficult aspect of having Lyme disease." Couldn't have said it better myself.

I have that sense of self-doubt even today, Borrelia. "I'm back! Wait, no, I'm not. Wait, what if it's not and never was Lyme disease? Do I have to start this roller coaster all over again? What's wrong with me and why can't I ever get well?" It never ends. And what about those feelings of isolation and of being misunderstood by family and friends? It's why I started this blog to begin with, Borrelia. I had to somehow let them into my world while venting to the world at the same time.

You're going to enjoy story time tonight, Borrelia. This Mad Bladder is going to start chapter 4! For more inspiration, more ideas, and more ammunition against your childish mind and body games! Good night, Borrelia in Wonderland.

The Lion, the Witch, and the Wardrobe

July 26, 2012

Well, Borrelia, I have a wonderful new friend. She reached out to me a few nights ago after reading our little blog, Borrelia. She too has been devastated by you. We talked and we connected. There is a reason we found each other.

The Lion. I shall call her Aslan, as in *The Lion, the Witch, and the Wardrobe* by C. S. Lewis. Yes, she is like Aslan because underneath the tiny sweet voice is a powerful lion fighting with strength and courage. Like Aslan, her life was "taken" from her until at last, a diagnosis and treatment plan slowly began bringing her back—just as Aslan was brought back to life.

Since 1997, my poor new friend suffered terribly with serious and odd symptoms, including blood in her spine, a brain bleed, and a hemorrhaged bladder. Most recently, she experienced paralysis of her arms. P-a-r-a-l-y-s-i-s. In the emergency room, they told her that the paralysis was caused by a deficiency in potassium. *Without even checking her electrolytes.* And later, doctors from one of Boston's finest hospitals sent her home and excused the paralysis away as virus associated. They then promptly ordered a psychiatric evaluation. If that doesn't make anyone feel like they are in a crazy fantasy world fighting for their life as Aslan did, I don't know what would.

The Witch. Obviously, Borrelia, you are the witch, the White Witch. In the series, the White Witch terrorizes Narnia. You, Borrelia, terrorize our anatomy, all of it. The spell cast by the White Witch is that Narnia is "perpetually winter, but never Christmas." Wow, I couldn't have expressed better myself what life can feel like with you, Borrelia. It can feel like an endless winter and without any Christmas. It's a feeling that in your world, the skies are gray, and you can't see the light. You can't even be sure if there is a light anymore. You can't be sure if joy exists. Or hope. Yes, *that* feeling: winter, but never Christmas.

The White Witch has special powers. She turns her enemies to stone with her wand. Borrelia, seems as though that is exactly what you have done to my new friend, turned her arms to stone. How dare you? For the love of Aslan, how dare you?

The Wardrobe. You are wondering how the wardrobe analogy comes in, Borrelia. It's quite simple. My new friend and I, we just *fit*. We both experienced an agonizing Lyme journey that left us tattered like old jeans. We suffered as moms, worried that we would not be well or alive for our kids. As we searched for help, feeling that we were dying physically, mainstream doctors told us we were psychologically not well instead. We now share the same Lyme-literate doctor. Interestingly, we share similar diagnostic results. We both had "indeterminate" results on our Western blot from IGeneX, the most reputable lab for this type of testing. Western blots test for the presence of Borrelia-specific antibodies as well as antibodies that might be present from other infections. The results for this test list a number of different antibodies and whether they are present or not. An indeterminate result for a Borrelia-specific antibody means that the antibody is present but not in a high concentration compared to a strongly positive result. So it typically makes the result "questionable" for that antibody and, therefore, "questionable" for a definitive diagnosis. But we also both had low CD57 results. As indicated earlier, CD57 cells are a subset of white blood cells that help fight infection. CD57 levels tend to be very low in cases of chronic Lyme disease. These results, combined with our years of mysterious and migrating ailments, lead our doctor to ultimately diagnose each of us with Lyme disease.

We share the same outlook as well. It is an attitude of gratitude. Yes, *gratitude* for finally having some answers and gratitude for not having some of the other conditions we were tested for. We have gratitude for finding the right doctor, having a treatment plan, and that our journeys have brought us together. And you know what, Borrelia? That makes me feel even more hope. For the both of us, like perhaps maybe our winter will have a Christmas. Or better yet, a spring.

Update: Aslan is none other than the brave and beautiful Kelly Downing, featured on the October 9, 2013, Katie Couric show available on YouTube. You can also get the latest updates on Kelly's courageous journey at 50ShadesofLyme.com and www.facebook.com/50shadesoflyme

Chapter 3

Mumma Mia!

***

Mum's the Word

August 5, 2012

Yes, having a mum and being a mum means being caught in the cross fires of worry. You worry about your child, and you worry about your mum at the same time. Right now, I can't even believe that the worries are converging; do my son and mum have Lyme disease? I recognize symptoms in each of them. Is Lyme disease pulling their strings like an evil puppeteer? Maybe I'm hypersensitive, projecting my experience onto them. Or maybe I am so in tune with Lyme that it's a sixth sense.

According to an article by Katina I. Makris, CCH, CIH, in the New England edition of *Wisdom of the Heavens, Earth, Body, Mind & Soul*, the CDC believes that there are over 300,000 new cases of Lyme disease each year and that only 10 percent of them are diagnosed. That leaves 270,000 undiagnosed cases. Partly to blame: inadequate guidelines by the CDC and medical professionals that are bound by these guidelines. Lab tests with error rates of 60 percent don't help. Climate change could also be a major contributor. Even in the Northeast, winters have become unseasonably warm, allowing ticks to "winter over" instead of die from frigid temps. As Ms. Katina points out, Lyme disease is a terrifyingly misunderstood epidemic that has exploded past HIV in terms of growth rate, making it the number 1 infectious disease in the United States.

For the past decade or more, my mum has struggled with immune- and joint-related issues. She is a complex case, and northern Maine rural medicine is not up for the challenge. The only diagnosis she has gotten from her doctors is "I don't know" followed by a lot of prescriptions to "treat" what they don't know. Inevitably, things only get worse.

At times, lupus, rheumatoid arthritis, other connective tissue diseases, and chronic fatigue were all considered possibilities. These are all things that you mimic, Borrelia. All the while, she has described burning sensations, tightness in her upper body, and allover pain. Because they have tested her for everything and essentially found nothing, she's been told, "It's most likely arthritis." Could my mum, who has spent infinite hours gardening in her yard and mine, have Lyme disease? Did you prey on her while she was giving the raspberry bush some TLC, Borrelia?

Am I finally the only one hearing what she's saying? We've even taken pause at some of the similarities of our symptoms, including the electrical-like sensations, burning feet, and tight, gripping pressure in the upper body. You know what I'm talking about, B. Recently, I told my mum that we need to find her a naturopath or Lyme-literate doctor. And that is at the top of my priority list, to help her do this.

Maybe it's just having Lyme on the brain, but I also wonder about my son. He was bitten by a tick in April. The tick was engorged and sent in for testing. As luck would have it, either the doctor's office lost it or never sent it in or the testing lab lost it after they received it. It was gone, Borrelia, and never tested. Therefore, we missed out on some valuable information. I opted not to have my son tested at the time. He was treated for three weeks with oral antibiotics.

Of course, I am on guard about any odd symptoms. So yesterday, when he presented with fever and chills and complained about arm and leg aches and back and hip pain, I couldn't help but be anxious about you, you bacterial bully. He had been in the sun. Yes, it was hot out. But something told me this wasn't heat stroke.

In the article by Ms. Katina, she describes how the life cycle of Borrelia is six weeks and how this creates a hide-and-seek-like effect on symptoms. Every few weeks, new symptoms can arise. What if this is arising now as a result of the earlier tick bite? What if it's taken a while for Borrelia to rear its frankenhead only to arrive now? Come out, come out wherever you are, this mama is ready to seek. Seek and destroy, that is.

I will be making him an appointment with my Lyme-literate naturopath. And God forbid, but if it's you, Borrelia, and not just a passing virus, I will make this the worst game of hide-and-seek in your life.

So, yes, Borrelia, I will go to sleep tonight worrying about my mum and worrying about my son. However, remember one thing, Borrelia. Make no mistake. I will never be mum, or silent, about you. I will talk, rant, educate, blog, whatever I can do to inform others and their families about you and how to protect and care for themselves as best I can.

Update: As of early 2014, my mum has not been tested for Lyme disease as she has been dealing with medical appointments for a broken hip. My son's test came back indeterminate, and his CD57 level was low. He was treated in August of 2012 as well as the summer of 2013 for several months. He is doing fantastic and has not complained of belly aches, headaches, eye twitches, or his hands and feet falling asleep since then.

The Levine Legacy

August 7, 2012

Borrelia, you and I hadn't even met yet when I met Margie Levine for the first time in early 2001. She was running a local chapter of the Institute of Noetic Sciences, a nonprofit research, education, and membership organization founded by astronaut Edgar Mitchell. *Noetic* comes from the Greek word *nous*, meaning "intuitive mind" or "inner knowing." Their mission is to support individuals and groups in awareness of consciousness, spirituality, and science to help in the realization of our innate human potential.

I used to love these meetings. There were always so many stories, mostly from women who had been through serious life and health challenges. And they were coming together to learn and harness the skills of tapping into their inner selves for healing. Part of this healing, as led by Margie, was visualization.

Margie was no stranger to health challenges. She wrote the book *Surviving Cancer* and was the longest survivor in the world of mesothelioma. Doctors gave her six months to live. She lived twelve years beyond that. Margie was so courageous and persistent that she convinced Brigham and Women's Hospital to adopt a new chemotherapy treatment protocol she had discovered while at Sloan Kettering Cancer Center in New York.

Margie lived a life centered on healing foods, exercise, nature, relationships, meditation, and maybe most powerful of all—visualization. Through visualization, it was as if she could intimidate her cancer cells. She would visualize the cancer in her body being destroyed or the healthy cells in her body taking over. I remember her telling me that sometimes she visualized her immune cells with jackhammers, pounding away at the diseased cells in her lungs. Visualization was a powerful tool in Margie's fight.

September 11, 2001, was the last day I saw Margie. It was a most beautiful morning, and we were having a chapter meeting at Margie's house. That day turned into one of the darkest of days as the terrorist attacks unfolded in New York City. After that day, for whatever reason, I never attended another gathering with the Noetic group. I never saw Margie again and learned of her death on the news.

I've been thinking about Margie a lot lately, Borrelia. I think that the concept behind Lyme Whisperer—of imagining and visualizing a dialogue between myself and a spirochete—was created in part as a result of what Margie had taught me. She taught me to use my intuitive mind and inner knowing to visualize and release the healing power within myself. Maybe these conversations with Borrelia are therapeutic as they allow me to expend negative energy and make room for the positive. As I visualize (and verbalize!) intimidating you and defeating you, Borrelia, these conversations free my mind and body—of the anger, fear, anxiety, frustration—so that the healing can begin. Without those negative energies, my immune cells are empowered to seek and destroy you, Borrelia. I know they are. I visualize those empowered immune cells as heat-guided missiles. And guess what, you are the heat source, the smoldering little fires all over my body that they seek to extinguish.

I wanted to tell you about this very special friend of mine, Borrelia. And I wanted to let you know that when I felt like the floor was rumbling like a train track today because of the vibrations and buzzing in my feet, I pictured taking a sledgehammer to the tracks and derailing the train. Then I pictured your evil little face under the conductor hat flying over the cliff as a result. It was a satisfying and empowering visual. I could just hear Margie laughing in the background. "Great use of visualization, Joy!" she would have said.

Thank you, Margie. God bless your sweet soul and everything you taught me. Life has a way of bringing people together for a reason, and now I know why I was meant to cross your path. Your spirit lives on, and I can visualize your smiling face.

PUSS 'n Hoots

August 9, 2012

Borrelia, today I am inspired by guest columnist Toni Bernhard of *Psychology Today*. I'm talking about part 2 of her article "What Those with Chronic Pain or Illness DON'T Want to Hear You Say." As Toni indicated in part 1, the purpose of her piece was not to make fun of those whose comments are off the mark (because, as she says, "Most people have good intentions"), but rather to help the friends, family, or colleagues of those who are sick to understand how some of their comments may be perceived. Her article shares examples of comments made to a person with chronic disease, followed by the thoughts and feelings of that person with chronic disease.

I laughed and nodded at the examples she gave. I could relate very well to the frustration and hurt. It inspired me to come up with my own sets of examples. I imagined a dialogue between what I will call a PUSS (**P**oor **U**n-**S**uspecting **S**oul) and the Lyme Whisperer (LW), all just for hoots. The PUSS in the examples below is simply making ordinary life observations. Lyme Whisperer is doing what she does best, responding with sarcasm from a Lymie point of view.

PUSS: My foot has been asleep for three minutes!
LW: My foot has been asleep for three years.
PUSS: Wow! That ride made me dizzy!
LW: Being awake makes *me* dizzy.
PUSS: I have a photographic memory!
LW: Memory . . . I forgot what that means.

PUSS: Wow, I can't believe how much these turnpike tolls cost.
LW: Wow, I can't believe how much the toll of Lyme disease costs. Let's see, doctors' visits, antibiotics, probiotics, vitamins, dark circle eye cream . . .

PUSS: I'm so tired.
LW: I'm so tired of being tired of being tired.

PUSS: I need a sugar fix.
LW: I need a body fix.

PUSS: Top of the mornin' to ya!
LW: Actually, mornings are rock bottom.

PUSS: Man, I really hate being in the limelight!
LW: Man (long pause), . . . I really hate being in the Lyme light.

Lean Mean Lyme-Fighting Machine

August 21, 2012

The Blood Sugar Solution, Borrelia. It's the most recent *New York Times* best-seller by Mark Hyman, MD. Great information on the book. A healthy lifestyle and more can be found at the website BloodSugarSolution.com.

I have known Dr. Hyman on a business level for a number of years and had the privilege of attending his book launch party in New York City earlier this year. Dr. Hyman's latest book attacks the issue of "diabesity" in this country. Diabesity refers to blood sugar and insulin dysfunction that leads not only to diabetes but to heart disease, cancer, dementia, and more. The book is an authoritative guide on the root causes of diabesity as well as the seven steps to regaining health by reversing or preventing it. How, Borrelia, how does this pertain to you?

For starters, *The Blood Sugar Solution* can also be considered the Borrelia Sugar Solution! You *thrive* on sugar, Borrelia, *thrive*. I think anyone affected by Lyme disease needs to take limiting their sugar intake *very* seriously. The last thing anyone would want to do, Borrelia, is to give you the edge. Sugar consumption in all its forms—evaporated cane juice, agave syrup, high fructose corn syrup—does that. *The Blood Sugar Solution* helps us realize that food in its whole and simplest forms prevents us from overloading our bodies with added or hidden sugars. Sugars, they are your little elixir of life, Borrelia.

Second, because Lyme disease is a chronic infection, the adrenals crank out cortisol, a hormone released in response to stress. In the case of Lyme, the body is in a constant state of stress from fighting the infection. Increased cortisol levels prevent insulin from working properly. As a result, blood sugar level increases and insulin resistance can develop. Lyme disease, then, could theoretically increase the likelihood of developing blood sugar problems.

Before being diagnosed with Lyme, my blood sugar levels started to show an upward trend. It didn't make sense. I had just lost twenty pounds from being so sick as well as switching to a gluten-free diet. Why, then, were my fasting blood sugar levels elevated? Once diagnosed with Lyme, my naturopath suggested that it was possible that the physical stress of the infection and my elevated cortisol levels were affecting my blood sugar.

The good news is that Dr. Hyman's new book provides those with diabesity and even those Lymies out there with issues like mine a road map to manage sugar intake, manage blood sugar, and optimize health.

What follows are the seven steps for regaining health as outlined by Dr. Hyman. I've chosen to embellish some of the points myself, with the Lymie in mind. What follows, if you ask me, are the steps for creating a lean mean Lyme-fighting machine—an Optimus Prime for Lyme, if you will.

Step 1: Boost Your Nutrition. Choose wholesome, simple, real food—not packaged, prepared, artificial, or processed. Eat lean meats and fish; grains like brown rice and quinoa; omega fatty acids from fish, flaxseed, olive, and coconut oils; antioxidant- and polyphenol-rich fruits like berries; and fiber-rich vegetables. Eliminate dairy, soy, and gluten if possible or if you suspect an allergy.

What I love about having read the book is that by following those criteria, I fell in love with great food again rather than eating to get by on a busy schedule. Avocados, herbs, garden tomatoes, rosemary-infused olive oil (drizzled on everything), coconut yogurts, fish, cashews, lemons and limes for flavor, nut butters, etc. It's simple yet satisfying eating. Maybe I wasn't able to follow Dr. Hyman's recommendation to the fullest and strictest sense. But I made simple changes that stuck.

Step 2: Regulate Your Hormones. This is important for Lymies. Cortisol is a hormone most likely elevated for most of us because of the stress of our infection. However, a diet high in sugar also increases cortisol. Yes, another reason to avoid sugar. And listen up, Borrelia babes, Lyme disease can really mess with other hormones, including progesterone and estrogen. I know my naturopath had me take some hormone-balancing herbs when Borrelia was messing up my menstrual cycles. Let's not forget melatonin, the sleep hormone. Many of us suffer from insomnia. Melatonin supplements can be a great way to get through this.

Step 3: Reduce Your Inflammation. Yes, this is a biggie, Borrelia, because Lyme disease *equals* inflammation. Inflammation makes symptoms worse. Inflammation also contributes to insulin resistance and diabetes. Sugar also contributes to inflammation. So again, Borrelia, we Lymies really need to get sugar out of our diets as much as possible. We are inflamed enough! Best to avoid inflammatory proteins—like those found in dairy and gluten—and consume anti-inflammatory oils and plant-based foods as mentioned in step 1.

Also, because of all the antibiotics we take, Lymies really need to minimize gut inflammation. My best advice for that is probiotics, which are healthy bacteria available as a supplement. They help eliminate bad bacteria in the gut and boost immune function. The one I took while taking antibiotics was VSL#3. Mind having a roommate in there, Borrelia? You shouldn't get along just fine. Haha! This brings us to step 4.

Step 4: Improve Your Digestion. In order to have a healthy gut, you'll need to eliminate bad bacteria, acid-blocking drugs like Prevacid and Nexium if you can, and food allergens from your diet. All these interfere with or damage the digestive tract. Take probiotics, enzyme supplements, and fiber to enhance your digestion. Repair the gut with omega-3 fatty acids and glutamine. Your naturopath or LLMD can help.

Step 5: Maximize Detoxification. In this section of the book, Borrelia, Dr. Hyman discusses how environmental toxins can make us fat. Toxins interfere with insulin and blood sugar. This leads to weight gain. Lymies need to keep their diet *and* their environment clean. Our overburdened bodies cannot afford to be overburdened with additional toxins. Choose natural insect and yard repellents; natural home-cleaning agents; natural skin and body products; hormone-free, antibiotic-free meats; and organic produce. Minimize exposure to acetaminophen or ibuprofen if it can be helped, practice moderate alcohol and caffeine consumption, avoid MSG, etc. At the same time, curcumin, silymarin, and broccoli extracts are examples of excellent detoxifying supplements that can be added to a healthy diet. A number of detox teas are also available. These support the liver, the body's primary detox organ.

Step 6: Enhance Energy Metabolism. Ener— what? Does any Lymie know what energy is anymore? Any energy we had now belongs to Borrelia. Or it is spent fighting this disease. I picture you aerobicizing inside of me, Borrelia, with a Richard Simmons headband and shorts, with all the annoying energy in the world. Well, we can try to reclaim ours.

Each of our cells has many little energy-producing factories in them called mitochondria. Mitochondria are most concentrated in muscle, the heart, and brain. When we face a chronic illness like Lyme or diabetes, our mitochondria don't function as well, and we face fatigue, exhaustion, and memory and cognitive issues. How do we keep the mitochondria churning and energized? Eating right (see step 1), enhancing protein intake, exercising, and considering supplement options like coenzyme Q_{10} and B vitamins.

Step 7: Soothe Your Mind. Dr. Hyman speaks of reducing stress because stress increases your blood sugar levels and therefore your likelihood of gaining weight and/or developing diabetes. He mentions techniques for stress reduction, including meditation, yoga, healthy relationships and friendships, dancing, laughing, etc. But Lymies also need to be connected and understood in order to soothe their tormented minds and bodies. That's why I built a community at LymeWhisperer.com. I also think in the case of Lyme disease, accepting the diagnosis—and most importantly the journey—brings a certain peace and healing that lessens anger, resentment, and frustration.

So to all my lean mean Lyme-fighting machines out there, maybe talk of *The Blood Sugar Solution* (or the Borrelia Sugar Solution) and the seven key steps to regaining health has been helpful. For Lymies, the idea behind the book in the context of our illness is not necessarily about fighting diabetes or losing weight. Rather, it is to get ourselves in fighting form. I believe these seven steps put us on the right path. I didn't read the entire book from front to back. I couldn't. I don't have the attention span or concentration level to do that right now. But I focused on what was important for me and hopefully for you too. Here's to our inner Optimus Prime. Let's transform ourselves and in the process defeat that Megatron Borrelia!

> **You Know You Have Lyme When . . .** the salesclerk at the store says, "Hey, sweetie. Didn't you buy the same dress last week?" and you say, "No, no, definitely not," only to find out she was right!

Leapin' Lizards!

August 25, 2012

"Leapin' lizards!" That's what Little Orphan Annie said. How about this for leapin' lizards? UC Berkeley scientists revealed that ticks that fed on the blood of the western fence lizard in California showed no signs of carrying the bacteria that causes Lyme. What? The implication of that is this: something in the blood of the western fence lizard, when sucked in by ticks, was able to *kill* Borrelia that lives in ticks! Meaning, the tick was no longer an infection risk to humans. Who is at the root of this great work? And what does this mean in the fight against Lyme disease?

Well, for starters, Dr. Robert Lane of UC Berkeley has a series of published works on this phenomenon. In Dr. Lane's 1989 study of 261 wild-caught lizards, there were no traces of the bacteria that cause Lyme in the lizards, even in lizards that had been bitten by infected ticks. In the 1990 study, Dr. Lane attempted to infect the western fence lizard with Borrelia and was unsuccessful. In the 1992 study, 0 of 223 tick larvae and 2 of 330 nymphs (0.6 percent) that had fed on the western fence lizard contained spirochetes. That meant that after the ticks had sucked in western fence lizard blood, any spirochetes the tick had once carried were dead. These results are only a partial summary, but they are impressive!

What does all this point to, Borrelia? It points to the fact that there is a borreliacidal factor in the blood of the western fence lizard! Borreliacidal—don't you loooove that term? *I do.* As indicated by Dr. Lane regarding his 1998 study, "We conclude that the blood of *S. occidentalis* (otherwise known as the western fence lizard) contains a thermolabile, borreliacidal factor—probably a protein—that destroys spirochetes in the midgut of *I. pacificus* tick nymphs."

A 2000 study shed some light on exactly that, that protein in western fence lizard blood may be by stating, "Proteins comprising the *alternative complement pathway* are responsible for the borreliacidal activity observed in the blood of *S. occidentalis*." Are there any other biology majors out there? In case not, let me break it down for you. The *complement system* is a part of the immune system that helps or complements the ability of antibodies and immune cells to attack harmful organisms in the body. It consists of a number of small proteins found in the blood, generally synthesized by the liver. These proteins typically circulate in inactive form until triggered. That means the complement system of the western fence lizard is triggered when exposed to Borrelia. And for some reason, the complement system of this lizard is effective in destroying the Borrelia when it is exposed to it.

Ironically, there is an eastern fence lizard, but this lizard does not show the same ability to neutralize the effects of Borrelia according to a 2007 study. Therefore, the eastern fence lizard does not help to reduce the risk of Lyme disease in certain geographical regions. Meanwhile, the western fence lizard *has* been shown to reduce the incidence of Lyme disease in the areas it is found in. That's because it is able to inactivate Borrelia in ticks.

Dr. Lane's most recent works were published in 2011 and 2012. After reading them, I had to wonder if studies were being conducted to isolate the protein from the western fence lizard or if anything was being done to develop it pharmaceutically or commercially. These could give us a potential therapeutic agent against Lyme disease. Well, why not ask the gentlemen behind it all? So I e-mailed Dr. Lane at UC Berkeley! Oooh, I felt almost as excited as Ralphie from *A Christmas Story* waiting for his Orphan Annie secret decoder ring in the mail. What would Dr. Lane say?

Unfortunately, this is where "It's a Hard Knock Life" comes in. Dr. Lane kindly responded by saying, "Thank you for your interest in our lizard research. Regrettably, we have nothing else new to report with respect to it since publication of our 2006 article demonstrating the refractoriness of the western fence lizard to *Borrelia bissettii* spirochetes. Again, thank you for contacting me, and keep up the good work."

Well, Borrelia, seems like us Lymies won't have a lizard potion any time soon. It's another hard knock for us. No vaccine. No magic pill. It's so disappointing that the western fence lizard may hold the key but nothing is being done, at least at the moment, to capitalize on this scientific discovery. Leapin' lizards. Here's to *still* holding out hope for our future.

Chapter 4

Getting 'Er Done

***

Twenty-Seven Ways to Get Stuff Done . . . When You Have Lyme Disease

September 3, 2012

I recently read a self-help article called "Twenty-Seven Ways to Get More Sh*t Done." This inspired me to come up with my own list of Twenty-Seven Ways to Get Stuff Done . . . When You Have Lyme Disease. Shall we begin, Borrelia? Here we go, in no particular order:

1. **Lose Five Pounds**. Ha. That's easy. Six antibiotic pills a day. Done.
2. **Make Dinner for the Family.** *Hmmm.* I'm good at shortcuts. Let's see, there is Paris night, which is a baguette, cheese, and grapes. Oooh lala, mama! There's nacho night, with tortilla chips and shredded cheese. Microwave on high for thirty seconds and you're finished. Way to go, mamacita! Breakfast night helps. Put peanut butter on those pancakes and you have a meal.

Make-your-own-salad night is a big hit at our house. Make-your-own-sandwich night. Make-your-own-taco night. See a trend?

3. **Clean the House**. Oh, that's easy. Strategically place fabric bins in every room of the house. All you need to do is throw sh*t in them and your house looks clean. Bins for school bags, bins for Wii games, bins for stuffed animals, bins for Legos, and bins for books and magazines! Bin there, done that!

4. **Entertain Your Friends**. My friends call me the Ten O'clock Tyrant. It's true. If you haven't left my house by 10:00 PM, I'm going to bed anyway. I don't care. I'm *tired*. Well, at least I tell them upfront. Like, "I love you, but you are outta here at ten. S-h-a-r-p. Leave the wine." Good thing they love me too.

5. **School Field Trips**. Fake it. Tell the teacher it's the kid who has to pee again, not you. And good lord, whatever you do, don't leave without the GPS. Your brain fog may be worse after a day with twenty-two four-year-olds and you want to get home *fast*.

6. **Playdates**. Playdates must always and only be at 10:00 a.m. That way they can play for two hours. Then it's lunchtime, and then it's time to nap with your toddler. This is perfect timing and the only way to get through the toddler years if you are a mom with Lyme.

7. **Work Trips**. Tell *no one* your exact flight arrangements or conference schedule. That way you can take a power nap when you need it or rest when you need to.

8. **Shopping**. Choose one store. If the clothes fit, buy several of your favorite items in the same color. This works for shoes, jeans, suit jackets, and slacks. I can spend five hundred bucks easy in a three-by-three section of Express. That's what I call efficient.

9. **Finish a Book**. Never mind. I can't help you with that one. I haven't finished a book in years. I'm always too tired and have too short of an attention span.

10. **Finish a Movie**. Oops. Sorry. I can't help you here either. I just can't stay awake. No *Avatar* or *Hunger Games* for me.

11. **Run a 5K**. Shuffle it. Walk it. Electric slide it. Just finish it.

12. **Help Son with School Project**. You know that birdhouse he built with his dad at Home Depot on a rainy Saturday morning? Cut a rectangular hole in the roof. Paint over the birdhouse. Now it's a second-grade Valentine's Day card box.

13. **Christmas Shopping.** Order on Amazon or get gift cards. And there is to be no wrapping whatsoever! Just bag it!

14. **Plan Daughter's Birthday**. That's what Build-A-Bear is for.

15. **Laundry.** Separate? Sort? Ha! That's funny! No, I don't think so . . .

16. **Clean My Office.** There is one file and one file only. File 13. Oh, looky. The desk is clean. The trash is full. Mission accomplished.

17. **Dictate.** Leave yourself voice memos on your iPhone. About all the sh*t you have to do. Or to buy grapes and cheese for Paris night (refer to number 2).

18. **Take Notes.** Forget the Post-its. Because you will literally forget where you put the damn Post-its. Take notes on your forearm instead. I'm serious. Write on your forearm with a pen. That way it won't rub off when you wash your hands.

19. **Go iPhone-Calendar Crazy.** This is a great way to remind yourself of everything! Doctor's appointments, birthday parties, meetings, girl's nights, work trips, medicine times, Dr. Oz, library book due date, hockey games. Imagine trying to store all this in a Lyme brain.

20. **Story time.** Nothing like having to read a pile of storybooks to two young kids at the end of a long day . . . unless you con them into a later bedtime *if* they agree to read to themselves.

21. **Host a Super Bowl Party.** Open red beans with can opener. Repeat with black and white beans, canned corn and tomatoes. Add prechopped onions and celery. Sprinkle with chili powder, then cumin. Turn on Crock-Pot. Touchdown.

22. **Walk. Like an Egyptian.** Yeah, exercise with Lyme hurts sometimes. But walk if you can, even with that pained, stiff, twisted, pinched back. Walk even if you look like an Egyptian. Exercising makes you fit, and being fit helps defeat Borrelia.

23. **Sit through a School Talent Show.** Bring your four-year-old. Then when you leave during the thirty-sixth act (with fifteen to go), blame it on *her* bedtime.

24. **Shop for Groceries**. Of all things, I think this one takes all my strength. I perimeter shop and keep it as simple and as quick as I can. I only dare to venture midaisle for the coffee, of course.

25. **Get Guiltless Downtime.** PBS, Animal Planet, Discovery Channel, History Channel. That's right, if you are watching educational stuff, you are learning, not resting. *Pffffft.* Everyone knows that.

26. **Quality Time with the Kids.** Let the couch games begin! I spy? Mother, May I? Simon Says? Charades? Taking movies with the iPhone? Yes, it can all be done from the comfort of the couch.

27. **Stay Sane.** This is a tough one. But find like-minded people. Or should I say Lyme-minded people? Is that an oxymoron? Do Lyme people still have a mind? Anyway, they are out there. Lyme support groups, blogs, Facebook communities. Find them because when you realize that you are not alone, you will not feel alone. And you will get more sh*t done.

See, Borrelia? We *can* manage to get stuff done despite all your pranks. Here's to all the Lymies who get it done or are struggling to get it done. Keep up the fight!

Dear Borrelia

September 26, 2012

Dear Borrelia,

I'm sorry. What part of "My kids are off-limits" did you not understand? Just now, after lying with my son in his bed, I thought, if only I could rid him of you by osmosis. If only I could make your spiral-shaped serpent self leave his body and get absorbed by mine. If only. And when I left his room, thinking of him alone in the dark, it tore me apart that you were in there, destroying him. You are a heartless, worthless grinch.

What a tough kid, behind those big green eyes and long eyelashes. Not really complaining much of the pins and needles, headaches, twitching, sleep disturbances, and belly aches. He just keeps playing ball and scoring hockey goals all the while. That's right. Indeed, the naturopath said today that he is fortunate to have my disposition and my genes, the defiant genes. The ones that say I will not let this get the best of me. The ones that say I will smile and laugh because I *choose* to be happy. The ones that say I feel sick, but I will push through anyway. Yes, those genes.

God, give me strength to keep a positive outlook so that I can help him do the same. Maybe this is why we met to begin with, Borrelia. Maybe God's plan all along was for me to get sick with Lyme first so that I could be his tour guide on the journey to the center of hell.

I used another analogy for him today. In a game that he likes to play on his iPad, he must fight an evil foe with a sword. And he earns points or money. With that money, he can buy potions. The potions give him an edge. He can mix and match his potions. He never knows which potion will best help him defeat the ultimate enemy. He must keep trying. Sound familiar, Borrelia? Using this analogy, I talked to him about antibiotics and how we will need to combine different ones to act like a potion. And that we might need to try different potions to defeat the ultimate enemy. You, Borrelia. We also talked about probiotics, homeopathics, tinctures, healthy eating, and exercise and how they are all part of the magic potion. Unfortunately for him, he has to play this game. Unfortunately for you, Borrelia, game on.

He loves Greek mythology. There are great stories and lessons and creatures and gods and heroes. Today, we read from his Greek mythology book, which came with a Zeus tattoo that he put on his forearm. Zeus was the most powerful god, the god with a shield and thunderbolt who defeated the Titans. Tonight, he is Zeus, and you are the Titan in this analogy, Borrelia. This is very symbolic indeed. And what about his sister? She chose the Pegasus tattoo, the beautiful horse with silver wings. Because despite all the fighting and bickering, she hates to see her brother hurt or in trouble and will fly by his side. I know she will.

So will I. I will be by his side with love, nurturing, understanding, a positive attitude, encouragement, tenacity, and at times, tears and frustration. But the end justifies the means. And soon, maybe you can be a myth for me and my family, a heroic story of our past. God willing.

Sincerely,
Lyme Whisperer

You Know You Have Lyme When . . . you fear the fire drill going off at work because your foot is dead asleep and any sudden movements to get up would mean falling flat on your face.

Lyme with the Wind

October 1, 2012

Well, Borrelia. How do you feel about some of Dr. Julia's patients starting an unofficial Lyme support group? We want it to be small and intimate, with meetings held at someone's home. We want it to feel more like a book club, and we want to brand ourselves. Sticking with the book club theme, we decided we should name our little group something with a literary twist. And why not go with a quintessential classic? And thus, *Gone with the Wind* becomes *Lyme with the Wind*. Our intimate little support group has been named Lyme with the Wind. Or is it Gone with the Lyme? Oh dear, it's Lyme brain at work again. But you understand, Borrelia. All of us in our little group do.

There is so much to weather with Lyme. Remission then flares. Emotional highs then lows. Progress then setbacks. Engagement then isolation. Complex protocols then treatment breaks. Somehow this wind has blown us all together, like destined little leaves. We met through our Lyme-literate doctor, and now we can weather the storm together. We can fight the powerful battle raging inside by standing by one another.

The powerful battle raging inside of us is not so dissimilar to the setting in *Gone with the Wind*. The story unfolds in Georgia, after the Civil War and during the reconstruction phase. Lyme disease is like having a civil war between our immune system and you, Borrelia. Think of all the ammunition and the diverse arsenal we must use. It seems enough to treat an army at times. We must also pick up the pieces and reconstruct ourselves.

Scarlett O'Hara and Rhett Butler enjoyed their life and privileges before the Civil War. But the war changed their lives forever. At times, we may feel like Rhett, Borrelia, "frankly not giving a damn." At other times, we may feel hopeful and persevering like Scarlett. "After all, tomorrow is another day," she said overlooking the cotton plantation in the closing scene, hopeful for her future.

As members of Lyme with the Wind, we can hope for our better tomorrows, just like Scarlett did, together. We can share our stories, the chapters of our lives, affected by Lyme disease. In doing so, we will learn from one another. We can trade battle secrets and strategies. We can support and reinforce one another. And someday . . . *someday* . . . perhaps our Lyme will be gone with the wind.

An Interview with Professor Polyphenol

October 3, 2012

A few weeks ago, in my blog post "Lean Mean Lyme-Fighting Machine," I discussed the importance of eating whole, fresh, healthy, anti-inflammatory foods. This week, I interviewed Kelly Heim, PhD, or Professor Polyphenol, as I like to call him. Professor Polyphenol will help elucidate exactly how polyphenols—compounds found in foods such as fruits and vegetables—can help our bodies defend against Lyme and other chronic diseases.

First, let's start with an introduction to this curious character, Professor Polyphenol. Dr. Heim is a pharmacologist who has just authored a chapter in a new book called *Antioxidant Polymers: Synthesis, Properties, and Applications* (Wiley and Scrivener). The chapter, entitled "Natural Polyphenol and Flavonoid Polymers," describes the pharmacology of polyphenols found in red wine, grape seed, cocoa, berries, pomegranate, and pine bark. I asked Dr. Heim for an interview to shed some light on the power of polyphenols and how we can make Borrelia suffer as a result. He was more than happy to oblige.

LW: Professor Polyphenol, tell everyone who you are, aside from polyphenol savant. Please tell us about your education, profession, hobbies, favorite color, pet peeves, or pets in general.

PP: I received my baccalaureate degree in nutritional biochemistry at UNH, the University of New Hampshire. By the time I graduated, I was entering the polyphenol world with tremendous enthusiasm and with a highly acclaimed review soon to be published in the *Journal of Nutritional Biochemistry.*

I went on to receive my PhD in pharmacology from Dartmouth Medical School in 2009. My favorite color is blue because it makes me envision anthocyanins, which are beautiful blue polyphenol pigments in berries and flowers. Please do not confuse this with the blue ink in pens. I have an aversion to blue pens, so I look around my office and kitchen junk drawer regularly to ensure my world is free of them. Blue ink aside, pet peeves include misplaced apostrophes and unapologetic distribution and sale of weak coffee. So far, over thirty cats, forty sheep, three parakeets, three dogs, and one lizard have been a part of my life. My hobbies include sports, art, writing, composing music, and handcrafting fishing lures. Places where you may run into me include university libraries, karate dojos, Banana Republic, batting cages, trout streams, and the seat of my 2006 Honda 225 cc 4-stroke dirt bike.

LW: Okay then! You've recently authored a chapter on polyphenols. Describe to the readers what polyphenols are, so as to avoid any confusion with Polly-O string cheese, which are great for kids' lunch boxes by the way.

PP: A reasonable request. First, let's take the word apart. *Poly* means "more than one." So polyphenol means more than one phenol structure. The example of a compound in nature with multiple phenol rings is ellagitannin, a polyphenol from raspberries. So polyphenols have more than one of these phenol structures hooked together. They can become quite large, with many rings and hydroxyl groups. This gives them antioxidant, anti-inflammatory, and antimicrobial activity.

Polyphenols are found in most fruits and vegetables, but Polly-O string cheese actually contains no polyphenols. But if you buy ten sticks of it, you can arrange them on a table to render the structure of a polyphenol structure. If you eat all ten sticks afterward and continue to do this several times each day, you will require more polyphenols in your diet to help offset metabolic syndrome from the accumulating paunch around your midline.

LW: Unbelievable. You are brilliant and sarcastic. No wonder why I like you so much. Realistically, not many of us will be picking up a copy of this new textbook . . . unless we go back to grad school for biochemistry or pharmacology (not going to happen). Simplify for us. Pretend you are writing a children's book on polyphenols. This is the kind of book we might be more likely to buy. What would the title be?

PP: I would call it *Let's Hold Hands.* A key point in the textbook chapter is that the types of polyphenols that are linked together in long happy chains are the hardest to measure and study, but we know they are extremely relevant to our health. Ultimately, I would like to see polyphenol intake incorporated as part of dietary assessment software platforms used in dietetics because high intake is relevant to long-term wellness. I would also like to support learning and visibility of polyphenols by mass-producing Christmas tree decorations to replace strands of tinsel and lights. Kids can string together chains of little plastic polyphenols and help put them around the tree.

LW: Polyphenol Christmas tree decorations. I didn't see that one coming. I like it. Now, why is it important that Lymies know about polyphenols and how to have a polyphenol-rich diet? I presume the antioxidant and anti-inflammatory activities of polyphenols is the key. Or should I say kiwi? Is there even any polyphenols in kiwi? Do you get the sense that you and I are easily distracted?

PP: Polyphenols have antimicrobial, anti-inflammatory, neuroprotective, and prebiotic properties that can benefit Lyme patients. There are over eight thousand different polyphenols known in the plant kingdom. They all have different properties and pharmacokinetics. Some are more effective than others for attenuating inflammation, quenching free radicals, enhancing immune function, killing bad microbes, and nurturing good microflora. Until all those relationships are defined, it is best to diversify your polyphenol intake.

The critical polyphenols are functionally versatile, and they are found in fruits and berries, certain nuts, the bran of grains, tree barks, certain kinds of beer, and red wine. Pomegranate contains a very different class known as ellagitannins, which are metabolized by gut bacteria to anti-inflammatory compounds called urolithins. Fruits, green tea, and red wine contain immune-modulating polyphenols known as flavonoids, which include quercetin and hesperidin. Kiwi will boost your intake of flavonoids. Resveratrol is a stilbene, a type of polyphenol that grape vines synthesize to kill fungus and bacteria in damp vineyards, and it does the same in your gut. Mix up and/or rotate your fruit and vegetable intake to make sure you are maintaining a diversified consortium of health-promoting compounds. By doing this, you build your defenses against the trashy spirochete Borrelia. Yes, we seem to be easily distracted.

LW: You just called Borrelia trashy. I think I love you. Design an ideal menu-for-a-day of polyphenol consumption, starting with breakfast. Include snacks, beverages, and supplements. But please, no pine bark. I just got my Invisalign braces off, and I am the Lyme Whisperer, not the Pine Whisperer, after all.

PP: Breakfast would be organic muesli or whole-grain cereal such as rolled oatmeal sprinkled with cinnamon, apples, and bananas or mixed berries. You could also include one cup green tea or dark coffee and/or eight ounces orange or grapefruit juice.

For morning snack, a handful of almonds and dark chocolate chips and a couple ounces of 100 percent Concord grape juice would be a great polyphenol boost.

Lunch could consist of salmon with pepper and lemon, mixed vegetables, and brown rice. A spinach salad with walnuts, dried cranberries, onions, and feta cheese with olive oil dressing would make for a great side of polyphenols.

Another square of dark chocolate, one-fourth cup strawberries, and a cup of dark coffee and you've got your afternoon snack.

Happy hour could include a glass of Pinot Noir. If you like the hard stuff, squeeze a flavonoid-rich lime wedge into your cocktail. Fresher limes are better sources of wonderful polyphenols.

For dinner, enjoy a lean meat of your choice, seasoned with some herbs and spices, steamed vegetables, and sweet potatoes *and* one more glass of wine.

Lastly, for dessert, I suggest a huge piece of blueberry pie!

LW: Sounds like a great plan to me! Seeing as polyphenols have a ringlike structure, is there any chance that this ringlike structure might serve to choke Borrelia if one consumes a polyphenol-rich diet?

PP: Borrelia is a long spiral-shaped bacterium known as a spirochete. The phenolic ring structure is, therefore, a geometrically suitable guillotine, as shown here:

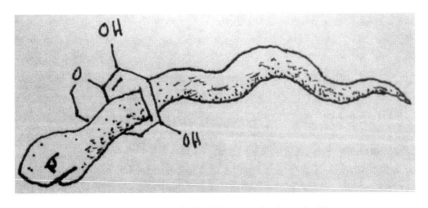

Borrelia getting choked by a polyphenol. Photo
Illustrated by Professor Polyphenol.

LW: Thank you, this is great. You are artistic, obviously. And I just happen to know that you like to draw lizards. Can you draw a lizard snatching up a tick with its long venomous tongue for the Lyme Whisperer? That would be so very gratifying.

PP: I most certainly can. How's this?

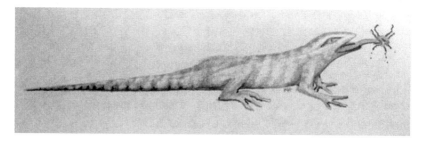

Venomous tick-licking lizard.
Illustrated by Professor Polyphenol.

LW: It's quite rewarding, actually. Is there anything you'd like to say to Borrelia while you have the stage?

PP: I am a native of Pennsylvania, where Borrelia has intersected the lanky legs of several Heim family members. Dealing with the Eagles-Steelers rivalry is hard enough, let alone the trash-talking spirochete that crashes parties in people's dermal layers. She needs to participate in the widespread undoing of her own crimes. I propose the formulation and manufacturing of an organic spiral-shaped polyphenol-fortified cereal called Borellios, to give her that purpose. She can pose on the front of the box in a swank little twirly dress.

LW: God, I love what goes on in that head of yours! Thank you for the interview, the inspiration, the information, and the oddball humor. We needed all of it! Readers can now follow you at DrKellyHeim.com!

You Know You Have Lyme When . . . you don't *really* care if the hometown hockey team wins. All you are worried about is getting an aisle seat so that you can deal with your Lyme bladder without annoying all of row M all night long.

Notes to Self

October 9, 2012

This week, I posted several "Notes to Self" on my Lyme Whisperer Facebook page. I've decided to keep that theme going. Here is a list of recent mental notes to self I've had to make:

1. Do *not* take your azithromycin and minocycline then skip breakfast, no matter how late you are for work. Don't do it. Your stomach just *can't* take it.

2. Not only should you not skip breakfast when taking your azithromycin and minocycline, eat *within five minutes* of taking them. Not ten. Five. Furthermore, you probably should not consume your Grande Bold from Starbucks too soon after the antibiotics hit the stomach. Ha! Who am I kidding? It's bold or bust, baby.

3. When your antibiotics have a tendency to upset your stomach, overeating creates the same discomfort as undereating. As in you will feel like hurling. Get it right. *Just* right.

4. Come on, girl. Pregnancy and morning sickness prepared you for feeling this way on your antibiotics. You know, feeling like you have the stomach bug for months. And doing everything you need to do despite it. You've got this!

5. If you want the laundry clean, you might need to actually *start* the washing machine before heading back up those basement steps. And it's okay if you still need to check several times over the next hour because you keep forgetting whether or not you actually started it.

6. Your children probably have homework tonight. Stop staring at the dining room wall.

7. Do not use your children's homework notebooks to brainstorm blog ideas. (A) That ruins their homework, (B) the teacher might steal your ideas, or (C) the teacher might suggest you get therapy.

8. For the love of God, please try to get to bed before 11:00 PM. It has most likely been a long workday, and those 5:00 AM Wii dance workouts come early.

9. As a matter of fact, you need to change up your morning workout routine. The back pain is really cramping your dancing style.

Maybe you should spend more time on the elliptical. And don't even think about ordering P90X. Not happening. Not now.

10. Disregard what you said about getting to bed before 11:00 PM. Staying up for John Stewart and Stephen Colbert on Comedy Central is totally worth it. Especially when it's for laughs like the Rally to Restore Sanity and/or Fear.

11. Be patient with the weird dyslexic tendencies lately.

12. Respect your iPhone calendar a little more. If it is alerting you to a meeting or appointment, you should probably get off the couch and do something about it rather than ignore it.

13. Start packing for your Vegas work trip now, twenty-six days early. It will take you that long to get all your sh*t together.

14. This time, when your vertigo is acting up, instead of trying to "keep up" at the Venetian's Tao nightclub in Vegas, take that as a sign to leave. Do not have concerned coworkers have to escort you back to your room. Again.

15. Don't start something if you can't . . .

16. Boycott the holidays. You just don't have the energy, patience, or need for more lists, reminders, or errands. You cannot store it all in your Lyme brain. And you can't accomplish it all with your Lyme body.

17. Try to focus on one thing at a time. Finding yourself in the middle of a dozen half-complete tasks is really overwhelming. And I'm pretty sure the kids don't appreciate half a lunch at the same time that your boss doesn't appreciate half of a presentation.

18. There are skinny jeans, and then there are "antibiotic skinny" jeans. Don't get attached to your antibiotic skinny jeans. You will be taking your meds for all the wrong reasons.

19. The one-pound dark chocolate bar from Trader Joe's should be on the grocery list every week. No exceptions. Stop second-guessing yourself. Of course you need it.

20. Order the darn teasel root tea already. You promised you were going to try it. You could have been detoxified weeks ago.

21. Don't be nervous about your doctor's appointment on Thursday. You are doing fine. You have support. Chin up, be strong, have a good talk with the doc, and make some good decisions on next steps. You can do this.

22. Consider donating body to science. That'll show 'em. Proof of what Borrelia does to a body.

23. Don't donate body to science. That'll show 'em. Proof of what Borrelia does to a body. You'll end up in Area 51.

24. Do not write notes for your quarterly earnings call with corporate on your hand. Revenue, gross margin, and EBITDA are mostly confidential. Well, not mostly; they are. Don't tempt the cashier at the grocery store to steal a peek.

25. Write "Ode to Whisperers Two Hundred Facebook Likes Tribute Poem." Sometime before three hundred likes.

26. Continue to write notes to self. It's a good mental exercise. And any mental exercise right now is good.

Awake and Alive

October 18, 2012

I'm going to keep it short and simple tonight. Sometimes, the little things need celebrating. Tonight, I'm just happy about Boy Whisperer's progress, even though we are only about three weeks into his treatment. Are you disappointed, Borrelia? Fabulous, I'm glad to hear it. Thought you could compromise the activeness and happiness of my kid? Yet what you find is that he is rising above you. Atta boy, Boy Whisperer.

Remember our appointment last week with the Lyme doctor, Borrelia? During my appointment, she asked me how he was doing. I told her, as you recall, that I really only noticed one change after he started on the antibiotics. And that perhaps it was the kind of change only a mother might be attuned to. I told her I felt like . . . he'd come alive. Like something had lifted. My mellow, quiet kid had become an excitable, more boisterous version of himself, with an energy that I hadn't really seen before.

Today, a friend told me that his teacher made a similar comment about him at school. That lately, he seemed energetic, talkative, and animated. It's a nice feeling, Borrelia, to have these comments from his teacher validate my observations. More reason to celebrate and allow myself to think that just maybe, just maybe he actually does feel better. Maybe all this time, he's never realized how unwell he has felt because it was normal for him to feel blah with Lyme. Until now.

Allow me to illustrate with some examples, Borrelia:

Before Antibiotics: *How was school today?* Good.

After Antibiotics: *How was school today?* Oh my god, NECAP rocks! (Sidebar: NECAP is the New England standard testing in schools.)

Before Antibiotics: *How was hockey?* Good. Oh. And I don't want to go to practice Friday.

After Antibiotics: *How was hockey?* Um, *awesome!* Can you sign me up for goalie practice Tuesday night?

Before Antibiotics: *How'd you sleep?* Bad—I woke up at two o'clock again.

After Antibiotics: *How'd you sleep?* Good, Mummy . . . Does this mean I can stay up later?

And a trooper he's been. He's taken antibiotics, probiotics, vitamins, herbs, and mushrooms without any complaints. He's embracing all of it and doing great. So coincidence or not, I'm just going to allow myself to feel positive and confident that he is winning his battle, Borrelia. And for that, I'd like to dedicate a song to him.

He's only eight, Borrelia. But he loves this song: "Awake and Alive" by Skillet. It's such an appropriate message right now. I simply feel that he is awake and alive and just want to savor the moment. So here's to Boy Whisperer: "Awake and Alive" found at http://lymewhisperer. com/2012/10/18/awake-and-alive/.

Quirks for the Herx

October 22, 2012

Well, how about that, Borrelia? Look at some of the very helpful tips from whisperers on getting through a bad herx reaction. A herx reaction refers to a Jarisch-Herxheimer reaction, which can happen after Lymies take antibiotics. The reaction is called a herx reaction for short. A herx reaction happens when antibiotics kill off bacteria—that's you, Borrelia— which then releases toxins into the bloodstream and surrounding tissues. Lymies might notice an increase in their symptoms or report feeling flulike because of these toxins. Some experience harsh herx reactions, some experience mild ones, and others don't experience the reaction at all. A herx can also happen in reaction to other treatments, including herbal and dietary supplement protocols to kill off bacteria or boost the immune system. Thanks to all of you who contributed your ideas on the Lyme Whisperer Facebook page! Happy healthy herxing!

From Becky: I use detox tea to help with detoxing. It's by Yogi. For pain I take tramadol because it's anti-inflammatory and not a narcotic. It is a prescription. Also gabapentin helps a lot with nerve pain. Epsom salt or just warm baths, heating pads, sitting in the sun, sweating (if you don't have a PICC or port) are also many of the things I have used to help with pain and detoxing. Soy frozen yogurt is a comfort food and *dark* chocolate is helpful for sugar cravings and yeast control.

From Gina: I would eat plain Stonyfield Farm yogurt for my tummy. Or green tea for my dizzy spells. I also heard cat's claw works well. It is an herb that acts as a natural antibiotic, but I never took it before.

From Emily: Have your LLMD look into glutathione. It was helped me more than I can describe. The first time I used it I herxed, but the next day, I felt better than I have in my entire life.

Detoxing is essential to feeling better. Also, try out coffee enemas (Gerson therapy), detox teas, Epsom salt baths, DMSA, and fresh organic lemon juice in water. Myers cocktails are great too. I get my glutathione from Infuserve compounding pharmacy in Florida. The folks there are amazing and care about you getting better. It can be taken orally, as a suppository, or IV (I think there is a nasal spray too?). I have been told that the oral form is the least effective due to the molecules' size.

Glutathione is a naturally occurring amino acid that is made by the liver; those who are immunocompromised do not detox naturally and don't create glutathione. It costs around $15 for a single dose by IV and can come with vitamin B_{12} too. Everyone I know who has tried it loved it. Once a week is best, but even once a month will help! Also, a multistrain sixty-billion CFU probiotic is essential (refrigerated), B_{12}, and fish oil. Good luck!

From Cate: I heard Essiac tea is great.

From Kathleen: I've heard about infrared sauna (it's expensive though) being helpful, as well as activated charcoal.

From Deb: Prima Uña de Gato worked the best for me. It's expensive but works. Any other form of cat's claw doesn't work.

From Dedee: For herxing, I love Epsom salt/baking soda baths. If it's really bad, I take a gabapentin. Best thing ever! Puts me right to sleep, and I wake up feeling pretty good.

From Tania: Hi, I'm a new follower. Epsom salts for me too. Also, sarsaparilla was crucial for me, helped curb the herx of my herbal protocol. Any sauna is better than none. Infrared and ozone are both great, but going to a standard one at the gym if you have the energy also helps. Drinking tons of water helps me, and glutathione for sure.

From Pamela: Glutathione is great, and don't forget Welchol (a cholesterol-binding prescription that binds the Lyme neurotoxins out of your body) and my everyday favorite (*not!*)—coffee enemas! For reduced glutathione and a very yummy treat, pick up some NanoPro by BioPharma. My doc had me start taking this back in 2008 for other reasons, and I still to this day take one scoop in a smoothie or with a little bit of milk, making it like a pudding. It has the most delicious vanilla flavor. You'll never know it's a "medical food," and it has *a ton* of protein too. Yum.

From Sarah: I have had some put-you-down-on-the-ground herxing. I started teasel, Samento, ETS essence, astragalus, and more water than I shower with. I was doing great for the first five days. Now I am experiencing fatigue, could hardly keep awake at work, waking with bad-oh-bad cramps in my legs at night. And I wake every two hours to look at the clock. I am getting pain throughout my body. I do not take any pain meds as I am allergic to NSAIDs and Tylenol, not good for the liver in this situation. I oftentimes find myself soaked with sweat, and my skin is very dry. But hey, I am alive and can for the most part put sentences together. Well, sometimes.

From Julie: I'm taking magnesium daily to relieve muscle cramps and spasms. I take 1,200–1,500 milligrams daily. It works!

Way to rally and support each other, whisperers! Lyme Whisperer says whatever works for a herx (glutathione, herbs, dark chocolate, pain relievers, dark chocolate, tea, dark chocolate, baths, infrared, dark chocolate, smoothies, dark chocolate, sunshine, dark chocolate) is what you should do!

You Know You Have Lyme When . . . you forget about the toast in the toaster and your child (who also has Lyme) doesn't get breakfast—not that he realizes it because he forgets why he's sitting there and thinks he already ate breakfast anyway.

Chapter 5

Viva la Starbucks

***

Onward

October 30, 2012

Onward: How Starbucks Fought for Its Life without Losing Its Soul is a book by Starbucks CEO Howard Schultz. Did you enjoy this read, Borrelia? I certainly did. Mr. Schultz bought Starbucks in 1987 and led the company through 2000, when he stepped down as CEO after a very successful and profitable reign. In the seven years that followed, Starbucks lost itself. It lost its identity, vision, philosophy, and path. It was fixated on profits and growth rather than customers and products. *Onward* describes Starbucks's downfall as well as its rise again when Schultz returned as CEO in 2007 with the task of rebranding Starbucks. Rebranding and helping it find its soul again.

This book spoke to me on several levels, Borrelia. As a business manager, I am always striving to improve my leadership skills. And I'm always trying to improve the brand while preserving the founding philosophy. But it also connected with me as a Lyme patient. We Lymies must always push and fight onward. We must always fight without losing our soul. Having suffered with Lyme for almost three years now, I feel I most certainly have had to rebrand myself, out of necessity. I will never be the same me again. Many things about me will be the same. But some things about me will never be as they were. On the flip side, some things about me will be even better because I've had to grow as a person and find inner strength.

Just as Schultz left Starbucks as CEO, I feel that I had to leave my former self behind. Once I realized that I would probably never quite be my former self again because of Lyme, I was able to step back into my life with a new outlook. I had a new mission to rebrand myself. What follows is a look at how you, Borrelia, have inspired me to rebrand myself. Who am I today because of this illness?

I Am an Actress. You cannot see my pain. My illness is invisible to you. But it's an act. I cry when you are not looking. I smile when you are. I can yell *action* and put on a brave face. But when it's time to cut, I just might fall to the floor. I did not ask for this pain, Borrelia. But I will ask—no, I will beg—for someone to take it away. And that won't be an act.

I Am a Firefighter. I must put out fires all over my body as new symptoms pop up everywhere, anywhere, at any time.

I Am an Herbalist. I'm learning more about antimicrobial herbs and treatments than my education as a biochemist and certified nutritionist would have ever taught me.

I Am a Pharmacist. I certainly feel like one when I am dispensing my daily dose of six antibiotic pills into my pill case.

I Am a Dancer. I dance to "Just Dance" on my Wii. Movement simply moves me. It brings me joy and peace. I love moving despite the pain. I love feeling fit. I started dancing when I couldn't run anymore, and I haven't stopped since.

I Am an Iron Chef. Time and energy are scarce, but I can throw a meal together in seconds. Already-cooked rotisserie chicken or ham steak? Perfect. Veggie omelette? So easy. Steamed green beans and microwave brown rice? Also ready in a snap. A "meal" might sometimes mean a Vitamix smoothie. Or broth. That counts too, Borrelia. It does.

I Am a Fund-Raiser. I feel for anyone suffering from anything. I understand what it is like to have a chronic illness. I understand what it is like to be scared and tired. I understand what it is like to be sick and to have treatments. And I want to help them. If there is a 5K for it, I'll be a runnin' for whatever the cause!

I Am a Coach. Time with my kids is precious, and it can be so very hard to be present for them when I'm not feeling well. So when I can be there for them, it needs to count. If that means being the batting order coach for the T-ball team, I'm in.

I Am a Follower. Faith takes on new meaning when it is challenged and when you find yourself begging God for help. I take comfort in the meditation, music, stories, and people of my church. And I appreciate all of it more than ever. Sometimes I think this was part of God's plan. That he wanted me to experience Lyme disease, to grow from it, to become a stronger person, and to meet the people I have on this journey.

I Am a Blogger. Lyme has given me the need for a creative outlet and for a meaningful outreach. Becoming a blogger has been one of the most rewarding rebranding initiatives I have undertaken.

I Am a CEO. Yes, most of all, Borrelia, I am a CEO. The CEO of my body and of my life. I think that makes me the Me-E-O. That means I am in charge of me, Borrelia, not you.

I have rebranded myself because of you, and I am stronger for it. It's onward from here, Borrelia. Onward. I will fight for my life without losing my soul. Even if I feel that I have lost my former self. The new self is much stronger for it. Onward I go.

Ringling Brothers and Barnum and Borrelia Circus

November 27, 2012

Funny, Borrelia. I was *just* lamenting tonight about how my hectic work schedule, being the business-planning and budgeting time of year, was keeping me from blogging more frequently about another day in the life of Lyme. I have also been feeling uncreative and uninspired. And not feeling very spontaneous with my writing. I've been too tired for it. But then, the phone rings!

It's one of my closest, craziest girlfriends. She called to give me an update after an urgent phone call she made to me at work Monday morning. I will give her the alias of UnCrazyLady. I know that sounds strange given how I just described her as one of my craziest friends, but you'll understand shortly why that's the alias I give her, Borrelia.

The development was this. Her husband, also one of my dearest friends, discovered a tick embedded in his leg. After removing it, not quite intact, UnCrazyLady starts to feel the panic set in. Why shouldn't she? She's been reading my blog for months! Posts like "Mind Freak," "Dear Borrelia," "The Mad Bladder," and "Note to Self!" That's enough to give *me* a panic attack, and *I* wrote it.

Her mind was racing. Her husband provides the household income. What if he can't work? What if he can't help her parent? His alias will be InItToWinIt. Why? He's not panic-attacking. He's a Whole Foods-buying, organic-eating, raw-cooking, exercising powerhouse. He's strong, fit, lean, and extremely health conscious. He's confident in his health and his body and has good faith that he is in great fighting form. I completely agree. If, Borrelia, he has been exposed to you, he will be more than a worthy opponent.

UnCrazyLady called me for some quick advice. They were going to contact his primary care physician and wanted any ideas on how to approach the visit and concerns. I indicated that most likely they would give him one dose of doxycycline. They did. I suggested that she push for at least a thirty-day dose. And in the meantime, research Lyme-literate experts in the area to consult with after that. She did push. He was not given the longer course of doxycycline. The doctor told her that the one-day dose was the CDC protocol and that he was not going to prescribe the thirty-day dose just to "treat" her anxiety. Then he looked at her like she was crazy.

Whoa, buddy. *I* can think that my dear friend is crazy for reasons deserving of a completely separate blog. But *you* cannot—I repeat—*cannot* think my friend is crazy when it comes to her concerns and questions about this. She is most certainly UnCrazyLady. You, Doctor, are the crazily callous one.

Feeling somewhat defeated, she asked whether the tick could be sent somewhere for testing. The doc said no, that costs $600. She called Quest, and they told her it costs $198. The doctor had told her not to worry because there was no bull's-eye rash or flulike symptoms. He told her to come back only if he does come down with flulike symptoms because those are truly the only indications of infection.

Oh, really? I didn't think that was good advice. I never had flulike symptoms. I told her to be hyperaware for even small things or changes, like experiencing eye twitches, feet falling asleep, recurrent sinus infections, or headaches that seem to be more frequent than normal. I told her to note anything new as well.

Meanwhile, UnCrazyLady told me that she had contacted Lyme specialists at Massachusetts General Hospital and Tufts Medical Center and is waiting to hear back from them. Her fight for information, access, help, resources, guidance, and answers begins. It's like a circus. The Ringling Brothers and Barnum and Borrelia circus! I'm so sorry that you have a ringside seat now, UnCrazyLady. So sorry. I have a vision in my head of *Madagascar 3*'s Marty the Zebra singing and dancing to "Circus Afro."

Look out, Borrelia. UnCrazyLady is a spirited, feisty, all-or-nothing fighter. She will make a circus out of *you!* She will track down the people and answers she needs. I will be learning from *her* in no time at all.

It is a hard position to be in, we agreed. We both do understand to an extent that not every single tick bite can necessarily be treated. Can it? We get not necessarily having an extended course of treatment every single time one gets bit by a tick. My neighbor, for instance, has had three tick bites in the last few weeks alone! Does every incident mean that one should push for the full thirty-day treatment? I don't know. It sounds like an impossible and improbable task. We live in the Northeast. This is our reality. The moment we set foot outside, we know it could happen.

Even when my own child had a tick, I didn't bring him to the doctor right away. Or have him or the tick tested. It was the beginning of the summer. He could go through the summer with one bite or one hundred. I waited for signs. And at the first one, acted. There's no right or wrong.

These are difficult decisions we face or will face, and so will our neighbors, friends, and family. It's the attitude of many in the medical profession that makes this dilemma so much more difficult. There is a lack of compassion and understanding and an inability to respond beyond "this is what the CDC says." They are not ringmasters, in control of the circus. We have to be our own ringmasters.

InItToWinIt takes his one dose of doxycycline tomorrow, and I'll be thinking of him. I'm sorry he is an act in this circus now. Someday, the tables will be turned. We will make a circus of the unsupportive medical profession. We will make a circus of Borrelia. I swear we will, and I believe it. Awareness and advocacy will be the key. With UnCrazyLady in the ring now, our ability to make others aware and to be effective advocates just got better!

The Coow Woow Interview with Dr. Nathan

December 5, 2012

Nathan Morris, MD, is a board-certified family practitioner. He is a founding partner at Indian Creek Family Health and practices functional medicine at his satellite office, Good Medicine, in College Corner, Ohio. Dr. Nathan was a guest in town recently while attending the International Lyme and Associated Diseases Society (ILADS) annual conference held in Boston in November.

This interview begins at the historic Longfellow's Wayside Inn, in Sudbury, Massachusetts, where we have just ordered lunch for a fireside table of six. Dr. Nate has ordered a Coow Woow. Pronounced "cooh wooh," rhymes with yahoooo! Right, Dr. Nathan? The Coow Woow is America's first cocktail served at America's oldest inn. Yes, even George Washington stayed here. It's not the fire keeping Dr. Nathan warm. It's the Coow Woow. Bet it was the same for George.

LW: First and foremost, Dr. Nathan, it's my pleasure to reveal the exact Coow Woow recipe for this historic, might I say epic ginger-infused experience that you so appreciate. I mean, who knew you were such a history buff? Oh, wait, it's more about the brandy and less about the history, isn't it? Well, it's good stuff, and here it is!

To enjoy a Coow Woow, mix the following*:

1. Two parts white rum
2. One part ginger brandy
3. Pour over crushed ice
4. Stir
5. Strain
6. Serve in a cocktail glass
7. Enjoy the alcoholic spirits and the colonial spirits of the inn
8. Start talking and let the conversation roll! Isn't that right, Dr. Nate?

Dr. Nathan: Yes! Thank you for the Coow Woow recipe, and it is so great to finally meet all of you! I cannot express how grateful I am for your hospitality. I am stimulated and excited by our conversation. I mean, I get

---

* unofficial Coow Woow recipe taken from the Internet.

to nerd out with Kelly Heim, PhD! Thanks for allowing me the opportunity to visit you all. And I would truly love to help in any way with you and your son's Lyme issues. And of course I would be honored to contribute some sound advice for all the Lyme Whisperer followers out there.

LW: You are Coow Woonderful. And that's not the Coow Woow talking. And yes, readers, the Kelly Heim he speaks of is none other than Professor Polyphenol, featured in "An Interview with Professor Polyphenol." Dr. Nate, thank you. You are as sincere as you are funny, smart, and crazy. What do you have against mops, anyway?

Dr. Nathan: That's funny, LW. I take it you are referring to a previous comment I made about my practice. My practice is built upon the belief that medicine should not be a pharmaceutical-biased, disease identification model. Rather, it should be focused on identifying the cause of disease and repairing this cause rather than just treating the symptoms of disease. For example, if your sink is overflowing, which is better, a plumber or a mop salesman? In the same way, functional medicine strives to be the plumber and fix the sink rather than making money selling mops. It's with this belief that my practice, Good Medicine, was established.

LW: There will be no mops here today since you have licked that Coow Woow cocktail glass dry. And most importantly, there will be no mops used in your approach to treating Lyme or other chronic diseases. This is why I adore and admire you. Tell me, as the plumber, then, what *is* your approach to fixing a very sick sink that is clogged, broken, gurgling, leaking, rusted, and hardened with Lyme?

Dr. Nathan: LW, initially, it's *all* about the GALT and the gut. GALT stands for gut-associated lymphoid tissue. That's where immune activation, inflammation control, and healing take place. The GALT is actually a portion of the immune system located in the gut. Actually, 60–70 percent of immune tissue is in the small intestine and determines 99 percent of our immune response usually. This is where nasty invaders like bacteria can be stopped before entering into circulation. However, our gut can also be invaded by allergenic foods we eat, which causes the body to mount an immune response. The first thing I try to do for my patients is to get the gut and therefore immune system healthy.

LW: Oh, I GALT it . . . Get it? "I got it" . . . "I GALT it"? Anyhoo. I can blame my stupid humor on Lyme brain. But seriously, that is a solid and practical approach. You also say you can help your patients many times for no more than $2.50 per day. Is this how you do it? By supporting the

GALT before recommending many of the other items we typically find as part of a Lyme protocol, including Samento, Banderol, and Byron White herbal tinctures? If so, how *do* you support GALT?

Dr. Nathan: Yes, I strive to keep my cost for most patients at no more than $2.50 per day, when on a maintenance regimen, but when treating Lyme initially, this may go up to $5.00–$6.00 a day. It could be much more expensive, but by addressing the basics of gut restoration, then you can use less supplements to support the immune system. My recommendations for supporting the GALT are simple but effective and might include various combinations of the following: vitamin A, olive leaf, arabinogalactan, glutamine, fish oil, probiotics, curcumin, Artemisia, garlic, phytostanols, colostrum, and nondairy immunoglobulins. The whole idea is to help the immune system, specifically the GALT, become more active. The immune system can be a Lyme-kicking machine when you activate natural killer (NK) cells, specific cells within the immune system that fight foreign invaders. I do check CD57 levels in my Lyme patients periodically. But that is only after focusing the treatment protocol on supporting the GALT, to determine if the body seems to be clearing the disease better.

LW: Cool beans. How else?

Dr. Nathan: Well, speaking of beans, of course the right diet plays a *big* part in maintaining healthy immune function in the gut. Gluten-free diets and/or dairy-free diets bring significant improvements to many. Eating whole, unprocessed, organic foods is key. Allergenic foods, bacteria, and medications like antibiotics and NSAIDs can cause leaky gut. A leaky gut is like a leaky sink, creating a mess and even damage. My practice focuses on this kind of dietary and nutrition counseling. Does all this answer your question about how to fix the sink rather than buying a mop?

LW: Yes. But I'm hungry for more. Can you elaborate on the damaging role of gluten and dairy on the gut, GALT, and overall immune health?

Dr. Nathan: Think of it this way. Gluten causes damage and opens the holes in the gut. Gluten then gets through the cracks and leaks into your system, causing a leaky gut and inflammation. This can cause an overactive immune response as your body tries to kill the foreign invader, in this case gluten. Can I give you a little history lesson, because I am so inspired by this historic setting . . . and beverage? Historically, wheat had been 97 percent starch and 3 percent protein, and 50 percent of that protein was comprised of gluten. By the 1870s, hybridized wheat had been introduced, a wheat with a protein content of 26 percent compared to the

3 percent it was previously. That's almost a 900 percent increase in the amount of gluten. This superwheat made for better baked goods for the American palate. But it also made for leaky guts! And allergic reactions!

LW: Good thing George was not around for the hybridized wheat. History may have been changed forever had he had a leaky gut!

Dr. Nathan: Yes, it would have! Now, another point I need to make is that you need bacteria to properly digest gluten. Antibiotics, which many Lyme patients take, kill bacteria—even the good kind—in your gut. This, then, affects one's ability to digest gluten, making it all the more important for Lyme patients to avoid it.

LW: And what about dairy? You know, "gluten's number 1 hombre"?

Dr. Nathan: Yes, you are right, I do refer to dairy as gluten's number 1 hombre! Dairy, like gluten, is very hard to break down. Dairy is homogenized and pasteurized, which breaks protein down into inflammatory molecules. It makes for inflammatory milk! Raw milk is better but not for everyone. Of course, there are so many alternatives now, like soy, almond, and coconut milks. So much gentler on the gut and GALT!

LW: Hmmm. Would you say that Professor Polyphenol is your number 1 hombre? And are there any other gluten hombres?

Dr. Nathan: Yes, LW, Professor Polyphenol is definitely one of my number 1 hombres! Well, another gluten hombre that I spend a lot of time counseling my patients on is . . . sugar. In any form! You *don't* want to feed bacteria or yeast in your gut with sugar!

LW: Okay, next question, and going in a different direction. I recall you saying it is critical to know your environment and, specifically, your risk or likelihood of mold toxin exposure. Why?

Dr. Nathan: Mold toxins cause similar immune suppression as Lyme. Twenty-five percent of the population is sensitive to mold. I've treated Lyme patients whose immune systems were handling the disease just fine until their bodies became overwhelmed by exposure to mold. You can't improve your Lyme symptoms if you don't resolve underlying immune suppression due to mold. In fact, mold toxin exposure can also suppress CD57 numbers just like Lyme does, so if exposed to mold, your numbers will be down even if you are doing a good job with treating the Lyme. There are tests you can take and labs you can use to determine your exposure to mold toxins. They include the ERMI test from Mycometrics and EMSL labs, which tells of your home's mold burden. There are also genetic tests that tell of your vulnerability to mold exposure, which involves HLA DR testing from LabCorp, and then a qualified physician to interpret this test. It is discussed in Dr. Ritchie Shoemaker's book *Mold Warriors.*

LW: Thank you, very valuable advice! Actually, I was just at my naturopath's office yesterday, and she ordered the HLA DR genetic test for me! I will soon know if mold toxins are playing a part in my inability to make progress with my remaining Lyme symptoms despite treatment for several years. Speaking of valuable advice, what was the most valuable or exciting information you walked away with from the annual ILADS convention? How to get at those darn persisters in the biofilm? Rad cyst-busting protocols? What?

Dr. Nathan: I think the biggest thing I walked away with is that we must approach this disease as if we are playing cat and mouse with it, as it is very effective at hiding. This includes using cyst-busting and biofilm-busting drugs like Flagyl and Plaquenil, along with other antibiotics. It seems that Lyme does not become drug resistant like other bacteria, but instead, it becomes good at hiding by forming biofilms and cysts so that antibiotics cannot reach it. When the antibiotics are gone, then it reemerges if the immune system is weakened. This is why doing pulse therapy, where short antibiotic holidays are taken followed by short courses of antibiotics, may be effective in the long run as the Lyme thinks the coast is clear and comes back out to play. That's exactly when you want to hit it again with antibiotics.

LW: Okay, now on the flip side, were there any developments that you learned of at ILADS that disappointed or discouraged you in your quest to help patients?

Dr. Nathan: I don't think so. I realize this is a really tough disease that has numerous aspects that we have to address from many different angles. I think I was more encouraged this time, than previously, that more doctors are starting to put the puzzle together and are coming at it from different angles. I think the functional medicine approach will be key as we address all the issues that coexist with Lyme and actually help it manifest. Gluten, mold, heavy metals, poor sleep, excessive stress, and the list goes on in regards to what weakens the immune system and exposes us to active Lyme, with an unhealthy gut being one of the most important starting points. It is my opinion there are a lot of people with Lyme who do not manifest symptoms, and I think we have the most to learn from them. I suspect the unifying factor with these people is an immune system not compromised by the factors listed above. Antibiotics alone will not solve chronic Lyme.

LW: Dr. Nate, it seems that our immune system can be balanced and activated to sustain the fight with Lyme and keep Borrelia at bay. You have convinced me that one of the best ways to do this is to support the gut and the GALT. And I don't think I am doing enough to do that. I have not put enough focus on repairing my gut and supporting the part of the immune system that resides there. I assume this means you have accomplished your mission to get this point across to me? I also assume that you want another round?

Dr. Nathan: Yes—Borrelia can be suppressed and its impact lessened. And yes, it all starts with supporting the GALT. Now, as much as I agree that the Coow Woow is the most amazing cocktail I've ever had, I actually can't have another. It's just too powerful. Is this how the revolution was won? Or celebrated? Wow! Potent stuff!

LW: Thanks, Dr. Nathan. This world needs more brilliant, creative, genuine, passionate, spirited, dynamic, *gutsy* docs such as you. I thank you for your time and your work as a clinician and researcher. I understand now that your approach to treating many conditions and chronic diseases is to treat the gut first. And that this is how you approach your treatment of depression, fatigue, allergies, diabetes, and rheumatoid arthritis. The gut is where it all begins. Hopefully for many people suffering, it is also where it all ends, with your help. Cheers to you and everything you do. And cheers to the Coow Wooooooow toooooo! To learn more about Dr. Nate and his practice, visit GoodMedicineOnline.com.

The Avengers, Darnit

December 18, 2012

This is a very quick shout-out to some of the superheroes in my life. These ladies are the strongest and most enduring and persevering people I know. We came to know each other because we are treated by the same Lyme doctor. And we have since bonded, laughed, cried, and encouraged each other as our own special little Lyme support club.

A few weeks ago, one of us, K, was going through an especially challenging week. We all rallied around her. I couldn't help but liken us to the new Avengers, fighting Borrelia and fighting as a team. So I assigned each of them an Avenger personality, and then they assigned one to me. Here's my tribute to my superheroes:

B: B, you are as strong as iron through some of the toughest of tough times. You have been in and out of the hospital. And you have been dealing with the challenges of TPN (total parental nutrition) tube feeding and of not being able to eat. You are Iron Man!

P: You are the hot Scarlett Johansson chick in the movie—the Black Widow is it—with the great hair and kick assitude. Yup. That's you in a nutshell. Kicking Borrelia ass for so long and so hard, you are a most relentless fighter.

K: You are the Incredible Hulk. Because of your teeny, tiny physique, that is especially funny. However, we all know that you are as strong as the hulk on the inside! You amaze me, the way your tiny body can fight so hard. Although some of your bouts lately have been scary, I am not scared for you because you are so strong, mentally, physically, and spiritually.

L: I'd have to say Captain America for you. Because in your own words from the other night, the antibiotic PICC line was almost like a security thing for you. You felt like it was your shield from Borrelia. Now, you are realizing that without it you are still powerful! And brave. And a great soldier in this fight against Borrelia.

D: You are definitely Thor because you have been hammering and hitting away at Borrelia (think Thor and his sledgehammer) for so long and with such strength!

Me: P said I needed to be one too and deemed me the Wasp. The Wasp has the ability to shrink to a height of several centimeters, grow to giant size, fly by means of insectoid wings, and fire energy blasts. In her words,

P said I could definitely fly with all my energy and that I am certainly full of energy blasts!

We are the Avengers, dammit. We have all fought so hard this year, and fighting together has been a wonderful plus. Ladies, let's continue to avenge Borrelia together!

Chapter 6

Mirror, Mirror on the Wall

***

This Is Your Year, Snow White

January 2, 2013

Snow White. She's my sweet, spirited, beautiful friend. With dark hair and fair skin. Who lays paralyzed in a rehabilitation facility. Her body unable to move. This fairy tale starts with the evil queen tick, who dispatches her huntsmen—Borrelia, Bartonella, and Babesia—to bring down Snow White. And now she is literally paralyzed by their evildoing, her body in a slumber.

The huntsmen may think they have your body in their hands, Snow White. But they don't. Use this time to reverse this spell, this poison. Allow your slumber to replenish your immune system. Nourish your body, and use physical therapy to restore your strength.

Your dwarves surround you, Snow White. There's Itchy. And Twitchy. Buzzy (that's me!), Dizzy, and Chesty. And don't forget Tubey and Newbie. Your Lymie dwarf friends, Snow White. Our spirits combined are still dwarfed by yours. We surround you. Support you. Relate to you. Understand you. Believe in you. And we are here to hold your hand. And we will be here until you find your prince.

There *will* be a prince-like influence that will ultimately kiss your slumbering body awake. Who or what will it be? The kiss of a new medication? The love of your seven Lymie dwarves? The tireless, caring touch of your family? A special prayer? Time? A potion with all that combined? Something magical is going to happen. And your body will awaken stronger than ever. The poison was inevitable; that's the way the fairy tale goes, after all. We knew you would be faced with such trial and terror. The time has come where you must face the poison. But every day, every sleepy, slumbering day, the poison wears off. Because no matter how toxic it is, your spirit thrives as an antidote.

When the time is right, your slumbering body will awaken, amid forest and sunshine, among the animals and songbirds. And in your castle, the magic mirror will say that you are the fairest of them all. And your happily ever after, your road to ultimate recovery, will begin. Yes, it will. Because this is your year, Snow White.

Update: Snow White is once again Kelly Downing, the same Kelly that inspired "The Lion, the Witch, and the Wardrobe" in chapter 2. After arriving paralyzed at Greenbriar Terrace rehabilitation center in Nashua, New Hampshire, Kelly finally walked out several grueling months later. In addition to being on the Katie Couric show later that year, she was invited to be the voice of Lyme disease in Washington, DC. I knew it would be her year, despite the fact that it began with the terrifying paralysis. Whether she wants the role or not, Kelly has been chosen to represent Lymies; I know she has. She knows she has. And she continues to raise awareness and advocate for change, despite her continued courageous battle.

NDNR Interview of the Lyme Whisperer

January 27, 2013

What follows is an interview of me for the January issue of NDNR, a newsletter for naturopathic doctors. The interview is conducted by Mark Swanson, ND. He is someone I have had the privilege of knowing for almost sixteen years. He has been a great support to me, and I appreciate his offering me a voice in NDNR. The treatment plans discussed were the treatment plans at the time of this interview. Lymies, take note! In this interview I make my plea to the naturopathic community on behalf of all of us, letting them know that we need their help.

Here are excerpts from the interview, as conducted and written by Dr. Swanson.

"Gluten-Free Lyme Whisperer"

Interview with Joy Devins, patient and advocate, with Mark Swanson, ND.

This issue of The Expert Report™ is a refreshing reminder that healing wisdom and learning comes as much from listening to our patients as it is does from the science, knowledge and understanding presented by fellow ND's and colleagues, medical specialists, researchers and academics. Our special guest is Joy Devins—a New Hampshire resident, naturopathic patient and health advocate. At 37, she is a vibrant and busy working mother, a runner and athlete, nutritionist, and fills a top executive position with a leading nutritional supplement company. She also faces her own personal health "issues"—namely the dual conditions of gluten intolerance and Lyme disease.

Not surprisingly, she has met many other fellow "Lymie-Glut's" through her support outreach and blog, www.lymewhisperer.com. She knows she is no longer alone or feels isolated. She's found the voices in the dark and as a result has made lasting friendships and close healing bonds. Through a health partnership with her naturopath, she has been successful at turning her health crisis into a proactive health challenge that refuses to let her become a victim of her conditions.

As a result, she is winning this long battle of endurance, conquering new heights, and now offers inspiration and hope for others like her. Joy has agreed to share her patient story, and insights on her health and healing journey with revealing details of her medical history, treatment protocol and passion for advocacy:

What's your secret to staying healthy in the faces of Lyme and gluten intolerance?

Positive attitude is number one, good fortune is number two. When I was diagnosed with gluten intolerance, I adopted a gluten-free lifestyle from that moment on and never looked back. I never focused on what I couldn't eat, only on the many things I could. My diet is much more diverse and healthy now, and I don't miss a thing. I say good fortune because I have been working in the supplement industry for many years, have met many health professionals like yourself, and was very aware and educated on gluten intolerance already. Because of these things, it was more or less a seamless transition for me.

Lyme disease—not so seamless. Lyme disease is a debilitating, isolating illness. I spent several years with frightening symptoms and no answers. Once the diagnosis came, I was thankful for all the things it wasn't, despite the private hell that Lyme disease is. I knew I would be here for my kids, so I was relieved, grateful and ready to fight. My gluten free diet, physical activity, and knowledge of and access to all the right supplements have been paramount to my health. I even ran my first 5K for Team Lyme this summer, and I haven't stopped running since.

What came first, Lyme disease or gluten intolerance?

I can't be sure. I was diagnosed with gluten intolerance first. In fact, because of some of my

Lyme symptoms—tingling and numbness in the hands and feet—I was tested for celiac disease, which was negative. Then later I was tested for gluten intolerance, which came back positive. I adopted the gluten-free lifestyle, but the tingling never went away. Two years later I was diagnosed with Lyme disease.

How long did you have symptoms of each before they were diagnosed?

I have probably been gluten intolerant for most of my life. I've had psoriasis since early childhood. As an adult following a gluten-free lifestyle, my psoriasis is mild and at times has been in almost complete remission. Before going gluten-free, it was moderate to severe. Regarding Lyme disease, I had obvious symptoms for two years before being diagnosed. Looking back, there are some instances before then that make me wonder if underlying Lyme was to blame, including two very difficult pregnancies and recurrent back problems. I never saw a tick, and never had a bull's eye rash, fever, or joint pain.

Do you recall the tests performed?

I had the genetic test for celiac disease, which was negative. I also had salivary IgG and IgA which diagnosed the gluten intolerance. Regarding Lyme, I had a Western Blot, which was inconclusive, followed by a CD57 count, which was indicative of Lyme disease.

Are you surprised that many others have both Lyme and gluten problems?

No, not at all. I have met many fellow "Lymies" through my blog who were diagnosed with Lyme and are now on gluten-free diets. They described their Lyme symptoms as worsening, especially headaches and stomach problems, when exposed to gluten. A number of people indicated that their food issues did not stop with gluten, and that they gradually became unable to tolerate other foods as well.

I am also the founding member of a Lyme support group in my community. At our last meeting, a participant described experiencing allergies to new foods often, sometimes every 4 to 6 weeks (which coincidentally coincides with the Lyme bacteria life cycle). She has suffered with Lyme disease for 21 years and her only symptoms have primarily been food allergies. Another member described sinus infections and persistent environmental allergies as her most obvious symptoms.

What are your most common and most bothersome symptoms?

The nerves in my hands and especially my feet are constantly tingling, vibrating or pricking like pins and needles. I've gotten used to feeling like I'm short circuiting. I'm forgetful. I have muscle twitches all over my body. I have vertigo. I'm forgetful. My bladder is inflamed and spasmodic. Did I mention I'm forgetful? I need to write things down everywhere, and all the time, so I don't forget them. And I have to push through fatigue every day. But most of all, it's the back pain. Did I mention forgetful too?

How would you characterize your digestion and GI function before and after being on a gluten-free diet and Lyme therapy?

I was fortunate in that I really didn't have many GI issues from the gluten intolerance. My issue was mostly my skin, specifically the severity of my psoriasis. With Lyme, however, GI issues consume me at times. First, there's the antibiotic-associated diarrhea. Second, there's a recurrent flu-like GI distress. I have periods where I don't experience it, then periods where I experience it every few weeks. It's hard to say if it's a Herxheimer reaction from the die-off of treatment, or the Lyme itself.

Even though the GI issues are bothersome, I tend to worry more about the effect of Lyme on my blood sugar and hormone endocrine function. My fasting blood sugar and progesterone levels are higher now with Lyme than they were before.

How many physicians did you see before you found the right one?

I saw six specialists and ended up in the ER. I bounced from one doctor to the next for two years. My symptoms were dismissed by my primary care physician and the neurologist as being stress-related, once MS and a B12 deficiency had been ruled out. The urologist, optometrist, and ob/gyn also found nothing, despite the symptoms that brought me to them. I thought I was dying and no one could help me. And yes, all the while working and being a mom. Finally, I landed in the hands of a competent Lyme literate naturopath, one of the smartest and most intuitive people I know.

Can you share some of your naturopathic treatments, a protocol that works for you?

As with the Lyme antibiotics, the herbal or natural protocols change every few weeks or months, as you adapt your protocol to your symptoms, which tend to migrate with the bacteria. In my first year of treatment, I mostly used herbal tinctures containing garlic, licorice, and Uncaria as an example, to target the bacteria, along with a high potency probiotic. In my current second year of treatment,

I am taking a more potent form of Uncaria extract that's free of tetracyclic alkaloids (TOA), Banderol bark extract, olive leaf extract, and maitake mushroom to target Lyme. I plan to add Andrographis and resveratrol to this protocol soon. I also take homeopathics to target the co-infection, in my case Bartonella. I also take a teasel root tincture and a greens protein drink for detoxification. Lastly, I take systemic enzymes to help lessen inflammation and as a result some of my symptoms. In addition, I continue to take a high potency probiotic formula too.

Are you also taking antibiotics for these conditions?

I have been on various combinations of antibiotics for two years prescribed by my ND. I currently take azithromycin, 500 mg once per day and minocycline, 200 mg twice per day. These target the Lyme bacteria in its spirochete, or spiral, shaped form. In a few months I will start

metronidazole (Flagyl), an antibiotic that goes after Lyme in the cystic form, the form it likes to hide out in. I am hoping to come to an end to my antibiotic therapy within the next six months, but it could be another twelve months or more. We may decide that I will never reach a point of being totally Lyme free and discontinue the antibiotic treatment. At which point I'll maintain a natural protocol, probably for the rest of my life, to keep my health in balance.

Does it cycle in you, with good and bad days?

Again, it mostly all comes back to attitude. I try to make every day a good day, despite it all. Except when my bladder acts up! Then there are some definite logistical issues. I'm just so grateful for the health that I do have. I think that the gratitude and inner strength is what people "see" when they tell me I look healthy or good despite the Lyme. On my "bad" days I power through fatigue, vertigo, back pain and brain fog. My symptoms do tend to get worse or change in 4–6 week cycles, sometimes longer. Sometimes the worsening of my symptoms coincides with a stressful week, a full moon or with my menstrual cycle. My symptoms always get worse in the fall and winter, without the summer sun.

How do you get through all this mentally and stay motivated to follow your treatment plan?

To push through the physical and mental challenges every day? I'm a warrior for my kids! I want them to have a strong mom and to see me as nothing but. I also have a child with Lyme, and need to be a strong role model for him. My 8-year-old is also on azithromycin 200 mg/5 ml once per day and rifampin 150 mg/5 ml, twice per day. He also takes the Uncaria, Banderol bark, maitake, and probiotics. We go to the same ND for our Lyme. He is a hockey and baseball player on top of and despite it!

I have no choice but to be positive and persevering. I am lucky to enjoy my work, my colleagues and employees, and that gives me purpose every day. They would say I am a productive and effective leader that has risen and continues to rise above this challenge. That motivates me even more. I want to be an inspiration within the Lyme community, for being physically strong and fit. That is also a great source of motivation for me. Lyme has been a horrific journey, but it has also been a blessing. I wouldn't change anything for the strength I've found, the lifestyle changes I've made, the prioritizing I've done, and the amazing people I've met, especially my new Lyme friends.

What can the naturopathic community do to better support individuals dealing with Lyme and gluten sensitivities?

ND's can help us have a voice and can be our advocates too. ND's can aspire to be Lyme literate by joining ILADS, the International Lyme and Associated Disease Society. There are so many obstacles, controversies and dead ends for Lyme sufferers. We need more naturopaths to take a stand for us. This is the epidemic of our time, the stats are out there. I know this to be true firsthand from my blog, www.lymewhisperer.com. I have followers from all over New England and the Northeast US, Pacific Northwest, Missouri, Montana, California, Kentucky, Texas, Florida, Ohio, Virginia, Pennsylvania and more. Internationally, Canada, the UK, the Netherlands and Australia. All of them suffering with Lyme and many also with gluten intolerance. And so many of them with nowhere to turn medically.

In a few short years, I have gone from knowing no one with Lyme to many in my community alone. My doctor's practice has grown and expanded and moved several times to accommodate the explosion of new cases. I fear that we won't have the doctors we need to handle this epidemic. We need you!

This is my plea.

You have the podium . . . and we are listening.

Gluten intolerance will always be a silent struggle, but with diligent gluten avoidance it is quite manageable personally and socially. Chronic Lyme disease is a much greater struggle and needs more understanding, rightful recognition and medical acceptance. One needs not have had a bull's eye rash, fever, or joint pain to be a candidate for Lyme screening, contrary to what some medical establishments believe.

The medical community and insurance companies should expect that many months of treatment will be required for chronic Lyme. It's quite commonly "brushed off" as a psychosomatic illness that "developed" after the initial short course 30-day antibiotic regimen ends (and fails). So many chronic cases are faced with mounting medical bills for their ongoing I.V. antibiotic treatments because insurance refused to cover after 30 days.

When someone is diagnosed with other chronic illnesses the medical profession seems more resourceful and supportive. In contrast, a diagnosis of chronic Lyme disease means you more likely be shunned and not viewed as being seriously ill. It's frustrating. Why was the vaccine pulled so prematurely, and why can't it be brought back? Why did research at UC Berkeley on anti-borrelial serum proteins from the western fence lizard stop, without the chance to be developed into a treatment? There are so many unanswered questions obstacles, controversies and dead ends for Lyme sufferers. With more help and recognition, we can prevent other people from suffering our same journeys.

The naturopathic community is one of the few trusted places we can turn. We need you to take on the challenge of Lyme disease, particularly diagnosing and treating it. That's how you can help us most.

So when you go to a party, club or something and see someone eating crackers or pretzels—do you get like all wigged out, or stay OK with it and just keep dancing, tingling feet and all?

Ha! The pretzels and dip are hard. Oh my! Just bring on the gluten-free beer!

Dr. Swanson's closing comment: Thank you Lyme Whisperer! More than any other health care provider, naturopaths listen most and embrace learning from their patients. Many will strive to meet your plea, even as far away as here in the Northwest and beyond! The late and beloved Dr. Bastyr said, "It's not the doctor that does the healing, it's the patient." Joy, your healing journey with the inspiration and hope it brings to others is no exception.

You Know You Have Lyme When . . . you panic when you see that your daughter's betta fish is not in its tank. And then you relax because you remember you removed it to clean the tank. And then you panic again because you don't recall where you moved it to.

Ten Things I've Decided Not to Stress About . . . When It Comes to Lyme Disease

February 22, 2013

This entry was inspired by an article called "Ten Things I've Decided Not to Stress About" by Sarah Klein in a Huffington Post article.

1. *I've decided not to stress about* missing the Route 2 exit on I-495 no less than twice a week on my way to work. Because I'm . . . well, I'm not really sure what I'm doing. Spacing? Thinking? Not thinking? Daydreaming? Forgetting where I'm going? All of it? For all I know, the detour could lead me to the coffee shop of my dreams.

2. *I've decided not to stress about* my cold, cold hands, feet, and core, despite the fact that I spend entire weekends at hockey rinks, watching my kids' games. I will hold a hot beverage. Wear long underwear and ski pants, double up on socks, sit on a blanket, and stuff my pockets with tissue. And I'll focus my energy on the referees, er, uh, game.

3. *I've decided not to stress about* long days at work, especially ones that involve late business meetings and dinners. I'll enjoy a dinner that I don't have to cook. And have a hit of cappuccino before the drive back home.

4. *I've decided not to stress about* my coffee habit. In case you haven't noticed, I've talked about it in the last three points. I know, I know. I'm not doing my adrenals any favors. At all.

5. *I've decided not to stress about* not being religious about taking my herbs. The stress of not taking the herbs is far more detrimental than not taking the herbs to begin with. Besides, give it a few weeks and I'll have to change protocol anyway.

6. *I've decided not to stress about* forgetting my grocery list. I mean, we eat the same thing week in and week out anyway. How hard can it be to wing it? Wait, what did we eat last week?

7. *I've decided not to stress about* whether or not my Lyme brain can handle quarterly reports, presentations, and budget plans that are all due at the same time. I will learn to do in one week what used to take me one month by simplifying and prioritizing. And a little help from—all together now—coffee.

8. *I've decided not to stress about* my clothes never fitting and getting increasingly baggier because of meds. Being super busy and active helps

too. It's not like my heart will be broken if I need to go to J.Crew at the outlet mall . . . again.

9. *I've decided not to stress about* my dark under-eye circles. I'll brighten up my look instead. Highlights make everything better. They may actually make the world go round.

10. *I've decided not to stress about* the allover twitching and buzzing and fumbling over words. Honestly, it would feel abnormal *not* to have these sensations and frustrations. *That* would be stressful!

If I Die

April 16, 2013

After yesterday's tragedy at the Boston Marathon, I wrote this poem for my children. This is a departure from my normal content, but the emotions of this tragedy consume me, and this is my way of expressing it while delivering an important message as a mom.

If I Die

If I die
While I wake
At a marathon,
movie, or baseball game,
Know that I
Didn't die in vain,
Know that I
Died in freedom's name.

If I die
While I wake
At a concert,
fireworks, or parade,
Know that I
Didn't die in vain,
Know that I
Rejoiced in our country's praises.

If I die
While I wake
On a subway ride
To a meeting or tourist place,
Know that I
Didn't die in vain,
Know that I
Whispered liberty's name.

If I die

While I wake
On a jetliner, cruise,
bus, or train,
Know that I
Didn't die in vain,
Know that I
Revered the eagle's face.

For if I die
While I wake
Because darkness showed
its ugly face,
Know that I
Have no regrets or tears
For living my life
Despite my fears.

For if I die
While I wake,
Following my dreams
In spite of evil's sake,
I will have stared it down
And defended our freedom
With my brothers and sisters
Even as civilians.

And if you ever,
My dearest child,
Find yourself
Amongst the crowd
When darkness falls
And rears its head,
Unite as Americans
And light shall prevail instead.

If I die
While I wake,
I leave you now
This message to take.
Be not sad or afraid,
Live the life that God gave,
Remember my words and the power they bring,
And always, always let freedom ring.

Chapter 7

Different Strokes

***

Mickey Mouse to Borrelia: "OMG!"

April 28, 2013

On Tuesday, April 23, at 8:30 PM at Disney's Animal Kingdom Lodge, I had the scare of my Lyme life.

We had been driving that day, from Fort Lauderdale to Orlando, to start the Disney adventure portion of our vacation. After arriving in the afternoon, we immediately hit the pool where we went for a swim, sunbathed, and enjoyed the poolside games. We also enjoyed the resort grounds, which was teeming with waterbucks, antelopes, giraffes, and zebras! We refueled with a great African-themed dinner at the resort's Boma restaurant—excellent cuisine complete with an ice-cold gluten-free beer called Omission. Omission. If only I could omit you, Borrelia, if only!

We were winding down for the evening, chilling at the arcade, then the hotel balcony. This is where things started moving in slow motion. Slow. Agonizing. Terrifying. Motion.

I came in from the balcony to get the kids' pajamas ready. I bent over a suitcase and suddenly felt my leg fold from under me. It was a bizarre sensation. Almost as if my leg was melting. Oh, I thought. Something is terribly wrong, terribly. This slow, warm, numb rush slithered up my leg. I tried to shake it off. Then my arm was under the same gripping spell, and I fell to the floor, unable to move my entire left side. My neck and head soon succumbed. It was like weights were tied to me. I felt so heavy, and I couldn't lift myself back up. It was almost like a magnet from the room below was trying to pull me through the floor. I was in a puddle on the carpet, like the Wicked Witch of the West. But I am *not* the Wicked Witch! You are, Borrelia. You are the Wicked Witch of the west, east, north, south, and every direction in between. But I didn't know just yet that this was your doing.

I screamed out in disbelief of what was happening. "I'm having a stroke, I'm having a stroke!" I screamed out to my husband, banging at him on the glass door to the balcony. All the while, my kids were witnesses to the terror and panic. I thought I was going to die that night, in front of them. I imagined them flying back home without a mom. I pictured their precious faces having to look at my casket get carried off the airplane. I actually thought I might leave them motherless that night. I wanted to pass out, but I was so damned determined for that not to happen that I fought tooth and nail not to lose consciousness. "I can't believe this is happening," I cried. I can't believe it. All I wanted to do was end the day watching Animal Planet with my kids. Why was this happening?

The paramedics arrived. "Can you move your left foot?" they asked. No, I could not. "Can you lift your left arm above your head?" they asked. No, I could not. This was not looking good for me. They agreed they needed to bring me to the ER. At this time, Borrelia, there was nothing in my mind that pointed to you. I had been going about my life just fine. I had ended my Lyme treatments four months earlier. Sure, I still felt dizzy, buzzy, twitchy, and tired, but that was all stuff I considered "normal" in the maintenance phase of Lyme. It didn't occur to me that maybe you had joined our little family vacation in such a big uninvited way.

At the hospital, they immediately did a chest x-ray to rule out a blood clot in the lungs. Then they did an EKG, a CAT scan, and blood work. All the while, I just cried, sat, and prayed. I was devastated to think that I might have just had a stroke. I thought of all the neighbors, friends, coworkers, and family I'd have to tell, and I felt embarrassed, ashamed, and deeply saddened. *God, please let me make it through the night,* I thought. I won't leave my kids, I won't. "Why is this happening?" I kept crying out as my husband held my hand. I take such good care of myself. I'm in great running form, eat well, and do everything right. Why was my body failing me? The stress was going to kill me if another "stroke" didn't first.

The first round of tests all came back normal, which was an instant burst of relief. But I was admitted overnight for observation. They had ruled out a heart attack and major stroke, but I needed an MRI to rule out a TSI, a transient ischemic attack, or mini stroke. Dammit, I wasn't in the clear yet. Nor would I be for the next fourteen hours, which is how long it took them to get me the MRI.

I did nothing but wait motionless in my bed. I didn't watch TV. I didn't talk. I didn't sleep. I didn't eat or drink. I just waited. I saw three doctors. The first two casually dismissed me when I said, "I have Lyme disease." But the third doctor was like a Prince Charming. He was young, compassionate, and calming. And when I told him I had Lyme, he nodded his head in understanding. In *understanding*. "Well, then," he said assuredly and confidently, "this could certainly be in the realm of Lyme." I felt some of my stress, frustration, and fear slip away. Not only did he acknowledge Lyme as my reality, he acknowledged that it could be behind this bizarre episode. In fact, he actually seemed very curious and eager to get my MRI results to see if a mini stroke could be ruled out while leaving Lyme as an open question. God bless this kindhearted, open-minded professional. For the first time, I felt some hope. I called my Lyme-literate naturopath on her personal phone. She assured me that she had seen this type of relapse before and would get me back into her office to figure out our next plan of attack. God bless her too. I told her I loved her and hung up the phone.

MRI negative! MRI negative! By all indications, no mini stroke! I could have jumped up on my hospital bed and performed the Little Mermaid's Magical Voyage Musical right then and there! I was so happy and so relieved! I walked out of that hospital cursing Borrelia but, at the same time, thankful it appeared to be just that and nothing else! I was going back to the hotel to see my kids!

The next day we shook, rattled, and roller-coastered our way all over Magic Kingdom! We tamed Space Mountain, Splash Mountain, and Thunder Mountain! Sure, I was a little leery, weak, and dizzy. But I had to laugh, wondering if all this jarring, jostling, twisting, and turning on all the rides was going to shake Borrelia up all over my body and make things worse or scare it back into hiding? Ha! I didn't care! I didn't have a stroke, and I was going to have fun and enjoy and show the kids that Mom was tough and nothing was going to spoil our fun!

Okay, so maybe I overdid it just a little. The next day, I had to experience Hollywood Studios from a wheelchair. And during each show, when the lights dimmed, I wondered, is that me or the lights? Was I about to pass out? When the air conditioning blew on my legs, I wondered if it was the air or if I was going numb again. With each step, I wondered if I would fall. Yes, Borrelia. It's always hard to know with you. But forget you. I wasn't going to let it stop me, despite the fear and discomfort and dizziness and weakness. And by the way, Borrelia. Speaking of Hollywood Studios, I am the director of me. Not you.

And so, I have returned to NH to begin another workweek tomorrow. I await an appointment with my Lyme doctor next week. Here I go again. On that roller coaster of Lyme. Hey, Borrelia. Mickey Mouse called. He doesn't want to see your kind of wild ride at Disney World ever again. Ever. OMG!

You Know You Have Lyme When . . . you try to sharpen your son's pencil with the deer call sitting on his desk.

I'm a Grad!

June 20, 2013

I've done it! I've graduated! From I-Want-My-Life-Back High!

Just four years ago, I was a freshman entering Dr. Julia's office for the first time. I was tearful, petrified, and desperate. My health was failing me, a D no doubt. I wanted my life back. And it was Dr. Julia that took me by the hand and walked with me through the cold, lonely, dark halls of Lyme. She was with me all the while as I learned one painful lesson after another. She believed me when I said it wasn't all in my head. It was during this time that she set the foundation for my education. It was easy, really. All I had to do was trust her. And listen to her. And do what she told me to. And so I did.

My sophomore year was a trying one. It was marked by antibiotic cocktails, tinctures, herbs, vitamins, and more antibiotic cocktails. Such aggressive treatments, such minimal results it seemed. The headaches, twitching, buzzing, numbness, fatigue, confusion, bladder inflammation, and back pain all persisted initially. But I was a studious patient, so I pushed forward, methodically and diligently. I did everything asked of me by my trusted teacher.

In my junior year, as any typical junior might do, I played hooky. I got tired and irritated with having to comply with my protocols. I stopped taking the antibiotics. Actually, I stopped taking everything. It was a rebellion in a sense. However, I was to come back begging forgiveness months later. Borrelia was acting up, and we needed to put her into detention or, better yet, suspension. I couldn't do it alone. I needed Dr. Julia for that. Borrelia was as fun as a bad prom date, and I'd had enough. Soon, it was back on the antibiotics for a while more.

Senior year was my fourth year in this journey and such a milestone. After taking antibiotics and natural remedies my sophomore and junior years, I'd reached a B+ or A−. My new assignment was to take homeopathics and to maintain with whatever I felt I needed: vitamins, probiotics, herbs, etc. My progress had been significant and was now stable. Sure, I still buzzed and twitched and tingled. And struggled with confusion and memory. I've had isolated attacks and relapses here and there. But I'm not the awkward puny freshman I was when I first walked into Dr. Julia's practice. And I'm ready to join the rest of the world again. And a bit to my surprise today, Dr. Julia agreed. And she said very proudly that she was pleased with my achievements and success and that it was time for me to move on. She said she didn't need to see me as a patient anymore. I had done it. I had graduated from the hard knocks of I-Want-My-Life-Back High.

And so here I am. With mixed emotions. The new grad of I-Want-My-Life-Back High, moving on to

Oh-the-Places-You'll-Go University. Like any grad, I feel both excitement and fear about what life will be like in this next chapter. I will need to master the art of diet, exercise, supplements, and rest to keep my health up. I will miss my classes, or appointments with Dr. Julia, but we plan to reunite annually to trade dark chocolate bars and retest CD57 levels. I did it, darn it. I did it! We did it! We got my life back even if the Lyme or Lyme symptoms are not gone. It's about time I get to move on. And I'm going places!

It's My Runniversary!

June 25, 2013

Since last year, I estimate that I have run about 650 miles.

It all started last June with the Rosanne's Rush for Research 5K, which raises funds for triple negative breast cancer that are donated to Dana Farber Cancer Hospital in Boston. It had been my first time back to running after being sidelined with severe Lyme symptoms for several years. I was proud to have overcome so many Lyme hurdles and to be well enough to be able to run again. I was emotional at the thought of raising funds in Rosanne's memory. I never met Roseanne, but I met her husband when he was handing out flyers for the race. I was instantly moved by the love and devotion of her husband and kids. And it put everything in perspective. I may have had my struggles. But I was alive.

This past weekend, on June 23, my son and I ran in Rosanne's Rush for Research for our second year in a row, marking my runniversary! Since last year, we discovered that he also has Lyme. My Boy Whisperer. And since last year, we have been putting one foot in front of the other, taking one step at a time. And you know what? We beat our time from last year by thirteen minutes. *Thirteen minutes.* That was a year's worth of determination and progress showing itself for both of us!

Yes, it had been a whole year since my return to running! In the winter, I run with my thermals, sometimes double layers of thermals! In the summer, I hit the pavement at 5:30 AM on bright beautiful mornings before work. I loved the idea of running a 5K every day before work just because I could. It felt so victorious! And with these sore, tired, and Lymie muscles, each and every run felt like it was the first. No matter how much I trained, it didn't get easier. For a Lymie, running three miles is as much of an accomplishment as running a marathon. And I'm tough on myself. And I'm competitive and defiant. So I pushed. And three miles soon became five. Five became eight. And last week, I reached my personal best of ten miles!

Six hundred and fifty miles later, I crossed that finish line on Sunday. I also crossed another finish line last week. When my Lyme doctor told me she needn't see me as a Lyme patient anymore. I had progressed so much, and we had done what we could do. She set me free. I finally feel strong. And look strong. Dear God and dear ASICS, please let me stay strong.

There's no stopping me now. I love what my runs do for my physique and my psyche. I love losing myself in my music and my thoughts. I love the high and the victory I feel after. Happy runniversary to me! The modern milestone gift for a first anniversary is a clock. Perfect. I would use that clock to time my runs this year. And I will work toward that diamond (tenth) and pearl (twelfth) runniversaries!

The Perfect Storm

July 25, 2013

What *the hell* happened last week?

For starters, work stress had been building until it hit me like a forty-foot rogue wave. Second, Boy Whisperer's second exposure to Lyme made me nauseous with "see" sickness after spotting a bull's-eye rash on his arm. And third, posttraumatic stress from the incident described earlier in this chapter in "Mickey Mouse to Borrelia: 'OMG!'" had been flooding my thoughts. It was the perfect storm. The convergence of these three fronts over my Lyme-weakened nervous system created rippling effects throughout my body—twitching, buzzing, weakness, lightheadedness. And a state of panic that was quickly getting out of control.

It was not the *Andrea Gail* sailing into a stormy sea. It was I, the Lyme Whisperer, trying to stay afloat amidst choppy waters. I was desperately trying not to give in to the feelings of collapsing or passing out. I was trying not to capsize. You pathetic, disgruntled, and opportunistic little deckhand, Borrelia. I can't believe you would wait for me to be weakened by stress to crash over me like this. Wait, yes, I can. That's what you do.

When I arrived at work Monday morning, the panic was crippling. I couldn't breathe. I could not get oxygen. It felt like I was drowning in my office. Until I was rescued by a colleague who talked me through it and spotted me an Ativan. On Tuesday, I woke up in a panic again. And had the same exact experience at work that morning. By Wednesday, the third morning of panic, I sent out my Mayday. I called my doctor for some Ativan. I could not free myself from the whirlpool of panic I was stuck in. I could not break free from what felt like a powerful riptide of panic, sucking me in further and further from reality. I needed a life preserver to get me through the week. I was in a neurological tailspin. But wait, was it panic? Was it stress? Was it a stroke? Was it Lyme? All these thoughts flooding my dizzy mind only added to the panic.

The doctor took on the role of captain. He got to the root of the anxiety overload. Work stress? He prescribed a beach day. Kid has a tick bite? A month of doxy is the right direction. Posttraumatic stress from stroke-like event? Let's get a carotid ultrasound and rule it out. And here's your Ativan.

Okay, I could actually feel myself breathing again. Yes, the Ativan helped. Yes, my son was being treated, and that's all I could do. Yes, thank God, the carotid ultrasound came back clear.

I still have my sea legs this week. I'm still a little shaky, weak, and dizzy. But I don't need to send flares out for rescuing. Good for me. I survived the storm. Not even Sebastian Junger could write a chapter in the perfect storm of Lyme.

The Funny Thing Is

September 14, 2013

The funny thing is, even though I am no longer seeing my Lyme doctor, I still don't know if I can put Lyme disease in the past tense. My nerves still buzz and vibrate sometimes, but nowhere near as much as they used to. Is it active Lyme or long-term damage? Can I say I *had* Lyme? Or do I say I *have* Lyme still? I don't know, and it makes me feel a little unsettled. Can't help but feel nervous about what lingers beneath.

The funny thing is, it takes a village to treat a Lyme patient. Ever since I stopped consulting my ND, my other ND, an MD, and my chiropractor for the effects of Lyme, I miss them. I miss the security of the mini army behind me. And the bonds with people I could count on and trust.

The funny thing is, I still feel like I can't keep up. I can't keep up with things outside of my normal routine. I can't keep up with all my friends and social circles, with the kids' sports schedules and school commitments, with the endless business meetings. I get run down and sick so easily. Is it Lymehaustion? Or just the normal fatigue of a tired working mom? And why does it matter? Well, I feel I would push myself more if it's "just being tired." But if there's a chance it's Lyme's still lurking under the surface, I would be a little easier on myself.

The funny thing is, now I feel nervous about *not* having the constant vibrating and tingling sensations. They became a part of me. I don't feel normal now that they are mostly gone. Panic attacks for *not* feeling my symptoms? This disease is so messed up. It really screws with your mind!

The funny thing is, I've wondered if I should still belong to my Lyme support group. Wait, of course, I should. I love my courageous comrades and want to pull them up with me. Lymies past and present have a brotherhood and sisterhood. And more than "people in a support group," they are my *friends.*

The funny thing is, I should feel happy that I am like a wounded bird that has been set free from the regular medical attention of my Lyme doc, but instead, I'm scared of smashing into a window. Hard.

The funny thing is, I still have moments of sudden vertigo. But I'm not sure if it's real vertigo or me thinking about having vertigo that makes me have vertigo. Do you have vertigo just from trying to understand that? Sometimes I feel like I'm going to fall. Sometimes movements or motion around me make me feel off balance. This probably goes back to Borrelia gnawing through some of my neurological wiring! I have a hard time trusting my body, and I don't like it.

The funny thing is, I feel like a jetliner in a holding pattern. Why do I feel this way? Why can't I just boost the turbo engines and fly full speed ahead, leaving Lyme and all the "what ifs" behind me? Truthfully, for the most part, I can. It's just that sometimes my psyche needs some maintenance!

You Know You Have Lyme When . . . your morning coffee is a puddle on the kitchen counter and floor because you pressed start on your Keurig without getting a coffee mug out first.

The Funny Thing Is: Take 2!

September 15, 2013

Feeling a little more rested and kick-ass this morning. Therefore, allow me to take my thoughts from last night in "The Funny Thing Is . . ." and redo it with a bit more of my normal chin-up fighting attitude:

Last Night: The funny thing is, I don't know if I can put Lyme disease in the past tense.

This Morning: The funny thing is, sing it with me now. Na na na. Na na na na. Hey hey hey. Good-bye!

Last Night: The funny thing is, it takes a village to treat a Lyme patient. And ever since I stopped seeing my Lyme docs, I miss them.

This Morning: The funny thing is, oh my god! I get to hang with *my friends* instead of my doctors now that I'm feeling better! Wine Bar, anyone? Come on, girls, let's go!

Last Night: The funny thing is, I still feel like I can't keep up with other people and with life in general.

This Morning: The funny thing is, my life is *ca-razy!* Work, commuting, hockey, soccer, baseball, sleepovers, parties, friends, committees, school projects, Lyme activism, blogs, travels, running! How lucky am I to have so many great things and people in my life! Everyone deserves a break once in a while, but life is good.

Last Night: The funny thing is, now I feel weird about *not* having the constant vibrating and tingling sensations.

This Morning: The funny thing is, bahhaaaaaa, Borrelia! I win I win! Suckah.

Last Night: The funny thing is, I've wondered if I should still belong to my Lyme support group.

This Morning: The funny thing is, hey, peeps! See you Thursday! Can't wait!

Last Night: The funny thing is, I feel like a bird set free, but I'm scared of hitting a window.

This Morning: The funny thing is, I am a beautiful osprey soaring through the air, quite possibly at higher heights than ever before! I went into this whole thing as a frail and sickly little sparrow, and now look at me!

Last Night: The funny thing is, I still have sudden moments of vertigo. Is it real? Is it still Lyme? Is it permanent lingering effects? Is it my imagination?

This Morning: The funny thing is, I may have posttraumatic stress from some of my Lyme issues. But eventually, I believe the vertigo will be vertigone!

Last Night: The funny thing is, I feel like a jetliner in a holding pattern. Why can't I fly full speed ahead and leave Lyme behind me?

This Morning: The funny thing is, I am JetJoy at cruising altitude, baby. I mean, have you seen my running sneakers? Hey, Borrelia. Eat my exhaust. *And* my dust!

You Know You Have Lyme When . . . you'd rather leave your keys in the ignition of your car and risk it being stolen than risk losing your keys. Again.

Chapter 8

Chamber of Secrets

***

Hermione: The Heroine of Haphazard Lyme Hell

October 10, 2013

She's done it yet again. She's inspired me to draw on powerful analogies to describe her epic fight against Lyme disease. First, I described her as Aslan the Lion in "The Lion, the Witch, and the Wardrobe" from July 2012. Then, as Snow White in "This Is Your Year, Snow White" in January 2013. And now, how can I resist but to draw analogies from the Harry Potter series when on October 9, her chronic Lyme story was aired in an episode of Katie Couric show called "Lyme Disease, Daniel Radcliffe" to describe her two segments. I mean, that's almost too easy.

No. It's not an analogy featuring Kelly as the brilliantly resilient Harry Potter and Lyme as the evil Voldemort, the darkest of dark wizards. No, it's not that. Come on. Hop on the Hogwarts Express with me. Let me tell you Kelly's Lyme disease story in my eyes. And it will soon become painfully clear why she shares the spirit of Hermione.

Like Hermione, she was born to "muggles." Wonderful, salt-of-the-earth, ordinary, hardworking, loving folks who supported her unconditionally. In time, she discovered she was a "witch" with special powers. In Kelly's case, she was a kindred, God-loving sweet spirit with the ability to spread light into the lives of others, including her family, friends, and students. Hermione was sent to Hogwarts School of Witchcraft and Wizardry to utilize her gift, while Kelly used hers as a wife, mom, and teacher.

At Hogwarts, Hermione was sorted into Gryffindor, one of four groups the students were assigned to. Those belonging to Gryffindor were identified as being brave, courageous, determined, unintimidated, and fearless. Kelly is most qualified for Gryffindor. Ironic, isn't it, that the emblem for Gryffindor is a lion. Wouldn't be the first time I compared her to a lion, like Aslan. Thing is, Hermione did have one weakness: flying. Now, for Kelly, it has been a while since she's been able to drive. For now, I would say that like Hermione, she is not a good Quidditch candidate nor should she attempt the Nimbus 2000 anytime soon. But not to worry, soon she *will* win that world cup in the game of Lyme, and she'll be able to do all the flying and driving her heart desires. Can anyone appreciate right now how hard it is for me to spell Gryffindor so many consecutive times with my Lyme brain and Lyme fingers?

Then Kelly's life turned into a chapter from *Harry Potter and the Chamber of Secrets*. In this second book in the series, a vicious, frightful, dragon-like, snakelike ancient monster is released and begins to attack students in the halls of Hogwarts. Hermione is caught in its grotesque and powerful stare, petrifying her. Literally petrifying her. Into a rocklike state. Like Kelly being stared down—and petrified—by the unsightly beast Borrelia. It first started with her arms. Then weeks later, full body, stone-cold paralysis overcame her. Petrified? More like *petrified*. And how did Kelly overcome? Much like Hermione did. With the magic and compassion of her caretakers.

Hermione, that heroine. She was the driving force behind Dumbledore's Army, a secret study group for the Defense against the Dark Arts. She fought with her comrades, including Harry, Ron, and her teachers, in a series of battles, including the Battle of Hogwarts that brought an end to the evil Voldemort. Just like Kelly. Leading with bravery our "secret society" Lyme support group. Taking us through our battles while fighting hers. Kelly, that heroine.

If Kelly is Hermione in all this, does that make Dr. Horowitz Harry Potter, the lead wizard in the fight against Voldemort-like Lyme? Yeah. It kinda does. And is the general public unintentionally walking around like muggles, unaware of the wizard and witch warriors around them affected by Lyme disease? As in the books and movies, the muggles do not see things in the wizardly world. Not their homes, their castles, their secret places. It stands to reason then that they certainly wouldn't see their pain. Just like a general public of muggles would not realize the world of pain experienced by those with Lyme around them. But Kelly is helping to change all that. She's bringing the often invisible disease Chronic Lyme to the forefront by sharing her story and raising awareness.

Kelly, you are a heroine, like Hermione. A heroine of haphazard Lyme hell.

The Polar Express: The Bell Still Rings Part 1

November 18, 2013

I awoke on November 9 to a beautiful, sunny, crisp morning. By 6:00 AM, I was rushing out the door, bundled up with a jacket and scarf. From New Hampshire, I drove to the subway station a few miles outside of Boston. It was finally here—the Lyme Disease and Tick-Borne Illness Community Conference. I had registered weeks earlier and had been waiting with Christmas-like anticipation. What would speakers, including Dr. Horowitz, reveal? What would be uncovered? Unwrapped?

I boarded the subway to Boston's Massachusetts General Hospital where the conference was being held. The train was warm and quiet. I was in the company of only two or three others. The rhythmic chug and grind made me realize a journey had been set in motion. A journey filled with both excitement and uncertainty. I felt like I had stepped aboard the Polar Express.

For the last few years, it seemed as though I had been holding a one-way ticket to Destination Chronic Lyme. I started to lose hope and belief at times. In the movie *The Polar Express*, the boy began to question his belief in the magic of Christmas. When his belief was gone, he was no longer able to hear the ringing, jingling bells of the season. At times, I also no longer heard the bells. My hope and belief in a magical outcome and recovery from Lyme wasn't always there.

I almost didn't take the train that Saturday morning. It had been an exhausting workweek. My son had a hockey game that afternoon. And I would be meeting up with friends later that night. Could I fit this in? Did I have the energy for it? I wasn't so sure. But something told me I had to. In the movie, when the boy hesitates to board the train, the conductor tells him the train is headed north and that it was "the year to board it." So the boy hopped on. Something was telling me to board this train, that it was "the right time to board it." So I did.

What would I learn at the conference? Would it be my ticket back to health? Would I meet wise Lyme angels along the way? Or would I be derailed by more talk of Lyme controversies and politics? My mind was racing until the chug and grind came to a sudden halt, and the conductor announced the stop: Massachusetts General Hospital.

The Polar Express: The Bell Still Rings Part 2

November 20, 2013

I stepped off the train. I suddenly felt alone and nervous. I wandered into the courtyard of the hospital entrance. I meandered aimlessly through the halls until kind strangers led me to the conference location. The Lyme and Tick-Borne Illness Community Conference had a waiting list a mile long, and people lined up hoping to get in at the last minute. I was feeling fortunate to have locked in my spot so early.

Once inside the conference room, I was rejoined with a few of my Lymie friends. Together, we sat with childlike awe, like the young CGI characters in the movie when they arrived at the North Pole. CGI is the art of blending two visual worlds: realism and fantasy. And isn't that just what it feels like to be in a Lyme state of mind? And isn't that just what it feels like to be caught up in a political disease? Yes, it feels like being caught in a middle world between realism and a nightmare. But we are not CGI characters. We are real people with a real disease.

Dr. Phuli Cohan, the first speaker that morning, knows firsthand just how that feels. Dr. Phuli is a pioneering integrative medical doctor. Her medical experiences took her to New Zealand and Australia where she developed her passion for Chinese medicine. Dr. Phuli fuels that passion by combining both Western and Eastern medicine in her innovative Massachusetts-based practice. Dr. Phuli is no stranger to Lyme and the warped realism/fantasy conundrum.

Dr. Phuli's first message: you can overcome this trying disease with perseverance. How does she know? She overcame Lyme herself, even after an infectious disease doctor refused to treat her for babesiosis coinfection, forcing her to succumb to her illness and to sell her medical practice at the time. Even after getting buried under an avalanche of symptoms and problems—light and noise sensitivity, headaches, tendonitis, memory problems, number confusion, word block, and being diagnosed with "brain injury"—she still overcame.

How? As Dr. Phuli put it, she learned more by being sick in bed than in med school. And from her bed, her protocol for recovery included seizure meds, PICC lines, herbs, and pulsing her antibiotics (cycles of on/off/on antibiotic use). Dr. Phuli advised that everyone frequently ask themselves the question: "Are you still sick?" If the answer is yes, and your Lyme symptoms still persist, change the plan. But always focus on three main areas: *toxins, metabolism, infection.*

In addition to the toxins generated by herxing or by taking antibiotics, Lyme disease makes the body susceptible to *lots* of toxins. Toxins from mold, yeast, viral infections, strep, staph—and anyone else on this type of naughty list—are, well, more toxic for someone with Lyme. The inability to clear these toxins affects the whole body, including the brain. Toxins that get into the brain mess with hormones, emotions, and heart rhythm. Having toxins is like having coal in your stocking.

Dr. Phuli's Toxin Removal Suggestions

1. **Antioxidant Support**: melatonin
2. **Electrolytes**: matrix electrolyte solution
3. **Nutritional Detox Support**: Vitamin C, n-acetyl cysteine (NAC), vitamin B_{12} as methylcobalamin
4. **Cleansing/Heavy Metal Chelation**: bentonite clay, apple pectin, chlorella, Microsilica

Importantly, Dr. Phuli also indicated the importance of being tested for the MTHFR mutation, a genetic mutation of folate metabolism that affects your ability to remove toxins, make neurotransmitters, and that can negatively impact your immune system among a host of many other problems. She also discussed the need to limit or eliminate exposure to psychological toxins. This includes toxic people and toxic thoughts. In other words, don't let your recovery be ruined by any Grinches or Scrooges.

On the subject of metabolism, Dr. Phuli reminded everyone to support the thyroid and adrenals as these control our metabolic functions and are disrupted by toxins!

Regarding infection, she advocated that everyone be checked for viruses, parasites, etc., and address them.

For metabolic function and defense against infections, she recommends nutritional repletion with magnesium, zinc, calcium, vitamin K2, lithium, iodine, vitamin A, and vitamin D. Now *these* would make great stocking stuffers.

***

The bell. I could hear the jingling of the bell in the distance. The bell that you can only hear when you believe. And over it, I heard Dr. Phuli's concluding words being sung as softly as a Christmas Carol: "Remove toxins. Replace nutrients. Consider the role of genetics. Don't rush. Be persistent. Take breaks. Take your antibiotics. Take your herbs. It might take years. But you *can* do it." Fa la la la la, la la la la.

And now, us CGI character friends looked at each other, satisfied and inspired by the pointers and direction, the encouragement and motivation form Dr. Phuli.

Next, Dr. Richard Horowitz would take the stage . . .

The Polar Express: The Bell Still Rings Part 3

December 1, 2013

Dr. Richard Horowitz of New York has changed the lives of more than twelve thousand in his twenty-six-year career as a Lyme protocol engineer and now as the world's preeminent Lyme expert.

As in the holiday classic *A Christmas Carol,* he was the messenger of Lyme disease past, present, and future that day. In his hands, he held a vast book that was five-hundred-plus pages long: *Why Can't I Get Better? Solving the Mystery of Lyme and Chronic Disease.* It is an immense guide that presents complex Lyme and coinfection antibiotic regimes like mathematical algorithms. It's an exhaustive resource of proper diagnostics. But perhaps most of all, it is a gift of compassion for the Lyme community. And it teaches other medical professionals how to have compassion and perseverance in treating chronic disease.

I took notes as he began his lecture and introduced some of the main concepts of the book, a thirty-eight-item questionnaire, a sixteen-point differential diagnosis map, and emphasis on multiple systemic infectious disease syndrome (MSIDS). Of course, there was focus on treatments, including antibiotic combinations and *rotations* as well as herbs and supplements for immune function, toxin elimination, and antioxidant support.

In writing his book, Dr. Horowitz's goal was to provide the most complete manual and road map ever completed for diagnosis and treatment of Lyme and chronic disease, based on his life's work. And ultimately, to provide a road map that could help health professionals establish chronic disease clinics throughout the country.

The lecture left me exhausted and confused, with so many complex details and protocols. And that was my first impression of the book when I began reading it at home as well. I wondered how anyone might realistically be able to digest it all and make practical use of it. I wondered how I could ever read more than the first few pages. I'm a Lymie, after all, who can barely get through a *Time* magazine. I thought maybe this wasn't going to be as valuable as I had thought. Not only to me but, more importantly, to physicians who may also find it overwhelming to understand and implement.

And then—and then—I slowly started to unwrap it. In layers. First, one chapter. Then, another. And another. Not from start to finish. That would lose my attention and be too overwhelming. Instead, I selected a particular section or topic, wherever my interest or energy felt focused in the moment. And then I couldn't stop. Skimming, searching, going from chapter to appendix to index back to a new chapter. Now, I couldn't contain my excitement. Like Ralphie in *A Christmas Story*, decoding the Orphan Annie secret message. It was possible. This book, it truly allows for the decoding of Lyme disease.

I hear it. The ringing of the bell. The bell that can only be heard when one believes. I believe now. Jingle bell, jingle bell, jingle all the way.

Below is my tribute to the lecture and the book. It's called "The Twelve Days of Lyme Disease" to be sung to the tune of "Twelve Days of Christmas." Sing it with me.

The Twelve Days of Lyme Disease: A Tribute to *Why Can't I Get Better? Solving the Mystery of Lyme and Chronic Disease* by Dr. Richard I. Horowitz

On the first day of Lyme disease, my Lyme doc gave to me *Solving the Mystery of Lyme and Chronic Disease.*

On the second day of Lyme disease, my Lyme doc gave to me a thirty-eight-item questionnaire and *Solving the Mystery of Lyme and Chronic Disease.*

On the third day of Lyme disease, my Lyme doc gave to me a definition of M-S-I-D-S, a thirty-eight-item questionnaire, and *Solving the Mystery of Lyme and Chronic Disease.*

On the fourth day of Lyme disease, my Lyme doc gave to me a sixteen-point diagnostic map, a definition of M-S-I-D-S, a thirty-eight-item questionnaire, and *Solving the Mystery of Lyme and Chronic Disease.*

On the fifth day of Lyme disease, my Lyme doc gave to me a bell that still rings, a sixteen-point diagnostic map, a definition of M-S-I-D-S, a thirty-eight-item questionnaire, and *Solving the Mystery of Lyme and Chronic Disease.*

On the sixth day of Lyme disease, my Lyme doc gave to me biofilm-busting antibiotics, a bell that still rings, a sixteen-point diagnostic map, a definition of M-S-I-D-S, a thirty-eight-item questionnaire, and *Solving the Mystery of Lyme and Chronic Disease.*

On the seventh day of Lyme disease, my Lyme doc gave to me doxy and Mepron for coinfections, biofilm-busting antibiotics, a bell that still rings, a sixteen-point diagnostic map, a definition of M-S-I-D-S, a thirty-eight-item questionnaire, and *Solving the Mystery of Lyme and Chronic Disease.*

On the eighth day of Lyme disease, my Lyme doc gave to me supplements for toxins and heavy metals, doxy and Mepron for coinfections, biofilm-busting antibiotics, a bell that still rings, a sixteen-point diagnostic map, a definition of M-S-I-D-S, a thirty-eight-item questionnaire, and *Solving the Mystery of Lyme and Chronic Disease.*

On the ninth day of Lyme disease, my Lyme doc gave to me herbs from Byron, Buhner, and Cowden; supplements for toxins and heavy metals; doxy and Mepron for coinfections; biofilm-busting antibiotics; a bell that still rings; a sixteen-point diagnostic map; a definition of M-S-I-D-S; a thirty-eight-item symptom questionnaire; and *Solving the Mystery of Lyme and Chronic Disease.*

On the tenth day of Lyme disease, my Lyme doc gave to me foods for inflammation; herbs from Byron, Buhner, and Cowden; supplements for toxins and heavy metals; doxy and Mepron for coinfections; biofilm-busting antibiotics; a bell that still rings; a sixteen-point diagnostic map; a definition of M-S-I-D-S; a thirty-eight-item symptom questionnaire; and *Solving the Mystery of Lyme and Chronic Disease.*

On the eleventh day of Lyme disease, my Lyme doc gave to me glutathione for all my pain; foods for inflammation; herbs from Byron, Buhner, and Cowden; supplements for toxins and heavy metals; doxy and Mepron for coinfections; biofilm-busting antibiotics; a bell that still rings; a sixteen-point diagnostic map; a definition of M-S-I-D-S; a thirty-eight-item symptom questionnaire; and *Solving the Mystery of Lyme and Chronic Disease.*

On the twelfth day of Lyme disease, my Lyme doc gave to me my ticket back to health; glutathione for all my pain; foods for inflammation; herbs from Byron, Buhner, and Cowden; supplements for toxins and heavy metals; doxy and Mepron for coinfections; biofilm-busting antibiotics; a bell that still rings; a sixteen-point diagnostic map; a definition of M-S-I-D-S; a thirty-eight-item questionnaire; and *Solving the Mystery of Lyme and Chronic Disease!*

Merry Christmas to all. And to all, a good fight.

Chapter 9

Land of Zombies

***

World War L

January 11, 2014

World War Z: An Oral History of the Zombie War by Max Brooks is the frightful novel of a zombie outbreak. It is believed by some that the author's underlying message was about government incompetence. The film was produced by Brad Pitt's production company, Plan B Entertainment. In the novel and film, this zombie epidemic unravels the world, country by country, with fear, helplessness, and utter chaos. Just like World War L. World War Lyme. If only Brad Pitt had a Plan B for World War L.

In the book, the zombie outbreak begins in Asia and Africa. Meanwhile, the United States is anything but battle ready. Just like in World War L, where many in the government and medical community have not armed the country to fight Lyme. When a zombie battle breaks out on US soil, in Yonkers, New York, the result is disastrous because the current methods of warfare didn't work. This is analogous to World War L, where the current campaigns of attack devised by Lyme-illiterate medical establishments and tactics used by government agencies are proving ineffective for desperate Lyme civilians.

As the plot continues, countries from around the world develop more advanced plans to eradicate the zombies. In addition, the US government commissions an Education Act to educate all civilians on how to protect themselves. Where is the massive Education Act for World War L? It seems this is left to patient advocates rather than medicine and government. Patient advocates, the true soldiers of World War L.

Only when the US military changed their tactics did the world begin to successfully turn the tides on the zombie war. They used different weapons. They fought longer and harder. Is that not how World War L should be fought, with persistence, perseverance, and long-term commitment by patient, physician, and insurer? And shouldn't our medical sergeants have the right reconnaissance, or diagnostics? And the right arsenal of weapons, including antibiotics, herbals, tinctures, or whatever it takes for however long it takes?

After World War Z, humans had barely escaped extinction. And millions of zombies remained dormant on the ocean floor or in the coldest corners of the world. In World War L, we also face an enemy that may lay dormant in our bodies. Medical generals worldwide must strategize to defeat the evil spirochete and keep it at bay before humanity suffers more. Where are these generals? Where?

New York. Not at the site of the Battle of Yonkers as described above but rather Hyde Park. This is where Richard Horowitz, MD, can be found—the best infectious and chronic disease general the world has to offer. In fact, this general of World War L has indeed plotted and formed alliances with world leaders. The prime minister of France called upon General Horowitz to ask about joining forces to change the CDC criteria for fighting Lyme. In China, leaders reached out to Dr. Horowitz for collaboration in defending babesiosis, an ally of the enemy, Borrelia. And in Japan, experts needed consult on *Borrelia miyamotoi*, a samurai of a Lyme spirochete fatal for children.

World War L *is* being fought with emerging Lyme-literate heroes leading the way. There *are* worldwide alliances forming. General Horowitz's new book, *Why Can't I Get Better? Solving the Mystery of Lyme and Chronic Disease*, is the epic battle plan, the epic map for winning the war. Red alert, medical, political, and CDC zombies; the world is slowly pulling together to rise above you. Civilians educate with blogs, support groups, petitions, radio shows, awareness campaigns, and public testimonies. When the new military, led by General Horowitz and others like him, is able to change the way the medical community fights Lyme, the ultimate zombie of all, Borrelia, will fall. To the death, Borrelia. World War L will be fought to your death.

You Know You Have Lyme When . . . you could have sworn that the box you bought yesterday said "plastic spoons," but now it suddenly reads "plastic forks."

The 2014 O-Lyme-Pics

February 8, 2014

Every day with Lyme disease is an Olympic event. It's unpredictable, hard on the body, and a test of the mind. It's filled with impressive feats, exhilarating achievements, and momentous letdowns. Here's an O-Lyme-pic tribute to all the Lymies out there who know exactly what I mean! Below are some recent Olympic versus O-Lyme-pic events from my daily life:

1. **Biathlon versus Biathroom:** Cross-country? Shooting? I can't even get across town without this Lyme bladder acting up. The only thing I'm shooting for is a bathroom around every corner. It's no coincidence that this is *number 1*.

2. **Cross-Country Skiing versus Stair Climbing:** My legs burn just from carrying my laundry up the stairs. Just looking to get up one level, never mind cross-country!

3. **Figure Skating versus Figure Standing:** With this vertigo, every other step can feel like the triple lutz or triple Salchow. Who needs figure skating for that?

4. **Freestyle Skiing versus Freestyle Sleeping:** Last week, shortly after dinner, I fell asleep on the couch with the remote in my hand. Only to find the kids had snuck it from my grip to order movies for the next three hours.

5. **Ice Hockey versus Eyes Hockey:** Seriously. How many floaters can one have in one's eyes? It's like skaters constantly gliding across the ice, er, eyes!

6. **Luge versus Lose:** I win the gold for losing and misplacing absolutely everything I put in my hands. My keys. The peanut butter. My son's iPod. My daughter's library book. I'm luging—I mean losing—my *mind*.

7. **Ski Jumping versus Pee Jumping:** Pee jumping should not be confused with the biathroom event. The biathroom is a mad dash to the bathroom. Pee jumping is jumping and writhing while enduring bladder spasms and trying to hold your pee in. Sometimes the pain just makes you want to jump off a . . . ski jump.

8. **Snowboard versus Snow Chores:** Nothing is worse than back pain from Lyme . . . except back pain from Lyme *plus* shoveling

out of the deep New Hampshire snow. What I'd give to snowboard into the sunset.

9.   **Speed Skating versus Speed Talking:** There's an obvious disconnect between my racing mind and my verbal motor skills. My mouth just cannot seem to keep pace with my brain. Which makes me sound like a stuttering mess at times. Like now. S-S-S-S-Sochi!

In Fear of Fun

March 12, 2014

In fear of fun I live
For Borrelia will pounce
When I've exhausted my energy,
Every last ounce.
Dizzy and lightheaded,
Weak in the knees,
Numb and scared,
Unable to breathe.

Somehow "everyday" life
I can, for the most part, manage.
Exercise and commuting,
My job, cooking, and practices.
Homework and laundry,
Groceries and games.
More, more, more,
And more of the same.

But throw in anything on top,
Anything at all,
The balance is tipped,
Damn it all.
Like packing for vacation,
Let alone the trip,
For the added endurance it takes,
I am not well equipped.

Remember Disney World?
And the stroke-like attack?
Borrelia was at her finest
Though I fought back.
I'm in fear of fun now
For what it brings,
Fatigue, overstimulation,
And a body on the brink.

Business trips, business trips,
Long hours and days.
Jet lag and marathon meetings
Make for Lyme haze.
Drinks and dinner with colleagues,
That's mostly okay,
But night caps and parties,
That much fun? No, no way.

I fear the fun
For it means more of me.
More weakness, more fatigue,
And more panicking.
A prisoner in my body,
A prisoner in my fear.
Please, dear God,
Don't let me fall—not now, not here.

But it happened again
On my California trip.
As in the Tower of Terror,
The darkness hit.
And the floor it seemed
To come out from under me
Until I fell to it
On my hands and my knees.

So much for dinner and drinks,
Laughs and hollers.
A Lyme body is not designed
For after hours.
And please don't judge
When after a week of work
I cannot find it in me
To get together with the girls.

Luck I will need,

All weekend, no doubt.
Hopefully the kids' hockey tourney
Will not take me down.
A weekend away,
A lot to endure,
Fun, friends, and family,
I will need strength for sure.

And to Boston it is
The minute I get back,
Another work trip that week
To conquer and tackle.
Possibly more excuses
As to why I can't join in.
I fear fun, I fear fun,
The explanation is quick.

Us Lymies, we love life and friends
Just like the next person,
But please understand
Our body is our prison.
Don't make us feel bad.
Don't make us feel guilt.
Every day is a challenge
Because our bodies are off kilt.

In fear of fun I write
To make people aware
Of what goes on with us
Because I know they care.
I try to create understanding
Where there is confusion.
I try to describe our reality
So there is no illusion.

Anxiety, vertigo,
Neurological fray,
Sensory overload, weakness,

An unsteady gait.
Overtired, overwhelmed,
Scared to fall.
Thank you for understanding
When we fear it all.

Yes, we want to have fun
And join the group
Or the event or get together,
We really do.
We are not antisocial
Or unfriendly or a bore.
We fear the fun
And what Borrelia has in store.

For when the balance is tipped
And defenses are down,
There is no other sheriff
Than Borrelia in town.
Help me stay calm,
Help me walk and stand,
Help me let the feelings pass,
And always, always take my hand.

You Know You Have Lyme When . . . blow-drying your hair is a difficult task because your arms keep falling asleep.

Happy Antiversary

April 23, 2014

Happy anniversary, Borrelia! What a special occasion. It's the anniversary of our stroke-like date. The only thing I want to remember is to forget about it—an antiversary. It happened at Disney's Animal Kingdom resort on April 23, 2013, and I wrote about it in chapter 7's "Mickey Mouse to Borrelia: 'OMG!'"

So, dear Borrelia. Here is my antiversary card just for you:

To the unlove of my life,
Who continues to be with me every step of the way, dammit.
It seems like just yesterday
We walked the Florida sunshine together
Until you decided to be the horrific partner you are
And brought me to the ground
In a "stroke" of sheer evil.
Thought I was going to die in front of my kids,
But I'm glad I'm alive
To wish you a happy antiversary.

Things have never quite been the same
Since that fateful day.
My left side is weak and uncertain.
Posttraumatic stress
Has been the gift that keeps on giving,
Thank you, but no thank you.
Really I insist
That you stop spoiling me
With all your lame surprises,
Please and thank you.

We've been through thick and thin,
Good days and bad,
But I really wish I could just blow you a kiss good-bye.
I don't need your "gifts,"
So on our antiversary, remember that,
And though you may be in my heart and mind . . . literally,

You will never infect my soul.
I don't know what the future holds for us,
But I promise to continue to love to hate you
Forever and always.
Happy antiversary.

Love,
Lyme Whisperer

Workin' Nine to Lyme

May 25, 2014

Being the vice president of a company and having Lyme disease is a challenge, to say the least. But I've learned to turn my limitations from the disease into strengths so that my work doesn't suffer. Here is a top ten list of how Lyme disease has actually made me *better* at my job:

10. **Marketing Materials?** I make them more concise, simple, and to-the-point when I edit them. Because that's what my easily confused mind needs. The end result? A stronger message for the brand.

9. **PowerPoints?** I use images and more images. Because lots of text overwhelms. The end result? Engaging and easy-to-remember presentations.

8. **Business Plans?** I start with a pie chart. Cut it into four equal slices. Fill in each slice with a main objective for the year. The end result? Strategy simplified. Serve it up!

7. **Quarterly Calls?** I speak swiftly and am direct and to the point. I deliver what I need to deliver in thirty-five minutes instead of sixty. The end result? No-bull reporting on results, and I finish before I start to lose my focus and thoughts halfway through.

6. **Time Management?** Having a shorter attention span means I carefully plan each hour with something new to tackle. The end result? There's no more procrastinating; every little project gets touched!

5. **Organization?** Lyme mental clutter on top of regular mental clutter means lots of clutter. The end result? I've stopped piling papers everywhere (most of the time) or filing physical documents. I only file electronically, to keep my desk, my files, and my mind clear.

4. **Leadership?** Some days, pep talks and motivational meetings are *all* that I can handle doing. The end result? I invest more time and energy focusing on my employees and leading by example than ever before.

3. **Social Responsibility?** My level of compassion for those that suffer or have been through a significant challenge is at an all-time high. The end result? Helping to institute and shape my

company's corporate responsibility program and having that as part of my legacy.

2. **Financials?** Financials schminancials. I can't possibly retain all the numbers I need to in this brain. The end result? I don't focus on my financials and make everything I do about the customer instead. Seems to be working for the top line if you ask me.

1. And a partridge in a pear tree. Wait. What were we talking about?

Lean Mean Detox Machine

June 4, 2014

Dr. Mark Hyman, MD, has done it again, Borrelia. He's written another *New York Times* best-seller. Dr. Hyman's latest effort is *The Blood Sugar Solution 10-Day Detox Diet*. I wrote about Dr. Hyman's original Blood Sugar Solution book in "Lean Mean Lyme-Fighting Machine" back in August of 2012. In that entry, I imagined a sugar-free lean mean Lyme-fighting machine to be like the heroic and mighty Transformer, Optimus Prime. I discussed how fighting sugar cravings and sugar spikes was important for fighting spirochete sugar junkies such as yourself, Borrelia. Did you know, Borrelia, that there are over six hundred thousand food products on the market, and 80 percent of them have added sugar? Did you know that mice, given the option, will choose sugar water over cocaine water as it is more addictive? Dr. Hyman's book is full of food industry secrets!

Yes, I'm happy to report that his new book inspires me to be an even leaner, meaner Lyme-fighting machine! It's my favorite of all his books. I read it in its entirety on my way to a conference in San Francisco where I would have the opportunity to see Dr. Hyman in person. I wanted to make sure that I had done my research. I wish all the passengers that day on my JetBlue flight had had a copy to read instead of watching their television monitors.

While the book is positioned for weight loss, it's really all about toxin loss. And detoxification is so important to being a stealthy, healthy Lyme warrior. I also love that it's a ten-day challenge. I can commit to ten days, especially if it means ten days of agony and sugar starvation for you, Borrelia. Now *that's* sweet! Hee hee! I did in fact do a detox challenge earlier this year. I had headaches and was genuinely sad about not having coffee. But I did it. I don't think I lost weight, but that was not my goal. In fact, I tried to make sure I didn't because this Lyme body doesn't need the weight loss; it needs the toxin loss. So I was careful to make sure not to shed pounds.

My goal instead was to activate and prime my body's natural detox mechanisms with laser-sharp focus. I followed Dr. Hyman's two steps for detox success: out with the bad, in with the good. Simple yet clear and effective. Out with the bad was hard. Not hard because of lack of willpower. Will power comes fairly easy to me. No, it was hard because most everything has added sugar in some form or another—and it all had to go. Agave, brown rice syrup, honey—things in many of my "health food" snacks and beverages like bars and bottled teas had to go. I said time-out to dairy, as well as grains, even gluten-free ones, as part of this detox jump-start. Even beans had to go. And, of course, my Starbucks and Shiraz. This was the cleanest, meanest detox I had ever attempted.

At the same time, in with the good was fun and rewarding. I loved my new decaf mint morning tea, was very satiated with my breakfast of hard-boiled or scrambled eggs, and loved to make my mountain-high Mediterranean kale salads drizzled with extra virgin olive oil for lunch and dinner. I snacked on almonds and sunflower seeds and enjoyed veggie/berry/protein smoothies. I loved all the foods in the book that I read about that boost my detox pathways, reduce inflammation, improve gut function, and balance blood sugar. Therefore, I really enjoyed meals like my tofu, broccoli, ginger, cilantro, curry stir-frys and lemon/cucumber water! I also fed my soul with outdoor running, journaling, relaxation, and sleep. If I'm not mistaken, Borrelia, you also got to enjoy the in with the good supplements I took, including the multivitamin, fish oil, vitamin D, fiber, and magnesium.

Ah, yes, it's nice to take the time to transform like this. I will try to commit to these "deeper detoxes" several times a year, where I cut out caffeine, wine, and allergens other than just gluten. The rest of the time, I have a gluten-free and Mediterranean diet anyway.

Doing what's right for our bodies and families often does feel like a battle between Autobots (that would be Optimus Prime, or us health conscious consumers) and Decepticons (that would be Megatron, or the deceptive food industry). Case in point, in using Transformer analogies for this entry, I had to let go of the fact that *Transformers* the movie was promoted heavily by Burger King. In fact, if you are fascinated by big food and big government influence over this nation, please see the documentary *Fed Up* in theaters now (or read this book), which was executive produced by Katie Couric and features Dr. Hyman.

Thank you, Dr. Hyman, for transforming the way we think about food and health. I personally am a leaner, meaner Lyme-fighting machine for it—an Optimus Lyme.

You Know You Have Lyme When . . . you accidentally spray yourself with PAM grilling spray instead of OFF! bug spray.

Her Name Was Leslie

July 20, 2014

She pussyfooted in
From the humid New Hampshire night.
Into the elevator we went
As she breathed deeply and sighed.
"Are you here for the Lyme meeting?"
She asked in barely a whisper.
"Yes," said my friend and I.
"Let's all go together."

Her cheeks were flush.
Her eyes a somber blue.
There was no sparkle or shimmer,
Just a dull, drab hue.
"What is your name?" I asked.
She looked so familiar.
"Leslie," she said meekly.
I knew our stories were similar.

The elevator door opened
To the church basement hall.
Husband and wife, father and daughter,
Moms and friends, came one and all.
We sat in a circle,
Some eager, some reluctant,
Most there that night.
Had just been inducted.

Into the Hall of Lyme, that is,
So new to the journey.
They'd thought the roller coaster was over,
But have learned otherwise in a hurry.
Diagnosis was just half the battle,
It became painfully clear,
That the next set of challenges
Would bring as much turmoil and tears.

Her name was Leslie.
She sat silently stunned.
Her head started spinning
As the facilitator begun.
One at a time, from right to left,
Symptoms were listed, antibiotics too,
Around the circle we went
About politics and Western blot blues.

Her name was Leslie.
And she sank in her chair,
Overwhelmed and unprepared
For this type of chatter.
Coinfections and rashes,
Diet, studies, and doctors.
Herbs, probiotics, and protocols.
It all made for mental clutter.

Her name was Leslie.
Her turn had finally arrived.
After almost three hours,
It was now a quarter to nine.
She searched the air,
For the words she couldn't find,
For the sentences she couldn't string,
For the blanks in her mind.
She'd seen the bite
Next to her pregnant belly.
She'd felt such anxiety.
It had turned her nerves to jelly.
She'd overcome stroke-like episodes
And battled numbness and sweats.
She cried for her babies,
Worried about their exposure threat.

Her name was Leslie,
And I wish I could have said,

Leslie, please don't worry
Your tired pretty head.
I've had stroke scares and anxiety
Just like you.
I also had symptoms during my pregnancy
And worry my baby has it too.

She had finally shared her story.
It sparked much advice, well-intended,
But she was exhausted and confused.
Paleness soon descended.
I didn't like what I was seeing.
I knew where this would go.
Her heart was racing
And the walls would soon start to close.

She was having an attack.
I wanted to reach for her hand.
Please, Leslie, stay strong, I thought.
Don't give in to the panic.
But before I knew it,
She'd ran out and left
So swiftly and abruptly
I hadn't a chance to interject.

I wish I had chased after her
As I heard footsteps running above.
She was out the door and gone for good
Before I could give her a hug.
Her name was Leslie,
And I felt all her pain.
Please, Leslie, please
Come back again.

You'll find a home here,
I promise you will.
Or another group somewhere,
You'll need them still.

Don't be deterred
From finding your place
Among the others
Who have stared the beast in the face.

Her name was Leslie,
And I don't want her to feel alone.
Please, dear God,
Help find Leslie her home
Among supporters and cheerleaders
And listening ears,
Shoulders to cry on,
And smiles to allay her fears.

Leslie, if you are out there,
There is so very much to take in.
We've all felt like you have,
Too overwhelmed to begin.
If I could tell you one thing,
It would be this,
There are many people and places
That can help you feel uplifted.

Lyme support groups can help
If you find the right fit.
Search books, blogs, and Facebook
For Lyme voices and advocates.
Her name was Leslie.
She has a place in my heart,
As do all the Leslies out there
Just getting their start.

There's a new class of Lymie;
Those who've made it through the thunder,
Who can help the Leslies of the world,
Like me, the Lyme Whisperer.
Because once we've weathered the storm,
We turn and extend our hand

So that we can pull the next in line
Toward the shores of sun and sand.

Her name was Leslie.
I regret I didn't reach out.
Please, dear God, just lead Leslie
To the hand that will be extended to her now.

Chapter 10

Whispers of Hope

***

Best-Case Scenario

May 27, 2014

So, Borrelia. There you have it. This is the end of almost two years of conversations, observations, and revelations.

You've seen me lose my mind, my keys, and my ability to hold my pee.

You've heard me cry for myself and my Lyme friends, laugh at the memory of my memory, and panic over panic attacks.

You've witnessed me choke down the last of 2,300 antibiotic pills and countless herbal sludges while wishing for you to be choked by a polyphenol ring.

You've seen me fall to the ground, get back up, only to fall and get back up again, *again*.

But this is a *best-case* scenario story, Borrelia. Despite it all, I sent you packing your *suitcase*. I kicked you to the curb, at least mentally, so that I could push on with my life.

During this time of chronicling my journey, I commuted to work over 500 hours.

I presented twelve quarterly reports and business plans to corporate, endured over fifty business trips, used only two sick days, and was promoted not once but *twice*.

I completed sixty-four hours of continuing education credits.

I ran over 1,300 miles and did hundreds of thirty-minute elliptical and Wii dance workouts.

I cheered at over one hundred of my kids' hockey games and over fifty baseball and soccer games.

I've enjoyed fifteen girls' night outs and hosted the same amount of cookouts and kids' sleepovers.

I never let the laundry, dishes, or groceries go undone.

I never even let myself go undone. I made over my clothes and my jewelry to keep me feeling confident, productive, and eager to get out the door and into the world.

I stayed positive. I didn't Google Lyme disease symptoms, treatments, prognosis, or politics. I listened to my Lyme-literate naturopath only and did everything she asked me to do. I focused on me and me alone, not the worst-case scenarios that turn up in Internet search engine results.

Look at all that can be accomplished despite the silent suffering, Borrelia. I want Lyme warriors to know that they *can* push through with strength, resilience, determination, will—and humor.

Of course, they need to respect and honor their limits. They must get enough rest, relieve stress, and find creative outlets. They must find the treatments, diet, exercise plan, and emotional support that best suit their needs.

They must believe that their instincts and intuition will guide them to the right path for their recovery and wellness.

I am not symptom-free, and they may never be either. But eventually, they will find themselves in a place where they can maintain a delicate but formidable state of balance—most of the time. They need to revel in that victory and progress. And they need to enjoy it. And to own it.

They also need to know that they may never emerge again as their former selves. No, instead they will emerge as an even better, stronger person that has grown through the journey to realize their full potential.

And whatever they do, Borrelia, I hope that they never stop whispering. I hope that they continue to whisper defiantly to you, telling you that you will *never* stop them.

Because they too can be a best-case scenario.

Top Five Lyme Whisperer Borrelia Busters

August 3, 2014

Borrelia, before concluding this book, I wanted to leave my readers with the answer to the question "How did you get better?" which I am so often asked. In order to answer that question, I have created a series of five top five lists. These top five lists do not serve as medical protocols or medical advice in any way. They are merely simple outlines of what has worked for me that may offer potential ideas for readers to pursue themselves.

This chapter and the next several chapters provide top five lists for treatment, diet, exercise, resources, and affirmations. The first in this series is found below, the "Top Five Lyme Whisperer Borrelia Busters."

1. **Rotational Antibiotics:** I took combinations of two to three different antibiotics at a time, and those combinations changed every six to eight weeks. The different antibiotics targeted Borrelia as well as coinfections. Rotating antibiotics helps prevent antibiotic resistance while sneak-attacking the bacteria with different mechanisms of action. I rotated antibiotics for nine months, took a four-month break, and then went back to antibiotics for another four months. Don't ask me which antibiotics I took. I don't remember. And I was too sick to care.

2. **Probiotics:** These are beneficial bacteria taken in capsule form. They boost immunity and help maintain a healthy gastrointestinal system. I took them two hours apart from antibiotics. VSL-3 was the probiotic that was recommended to me by my Lyme-literate ND.

3. **Herbal Tinctures:** Herbs boost the immune system while providing antimicrobial activities. Samento and Banderol from NutraMedix, as well as Maitake Gold 404 from Mushroom Science, were indispensable to me. Byron White Formulas also played a role.

4. **Supplements:** I boosted my health with supplements throughout my journey. I took liposomal glutathione for antioxidant and

detoxification support; olive leaf, vitamin D, and n-acetyl cysteine for immune defense; magnesium for muscle spasms and weakness; and B complex and adrenal support formulas for energy, to name a few. Now, I maintain my health with a multivitamin, vitamin D, and probiotics.

5. **Homeopathics:** Deseret Biologicals offers a Borrelia series homeopathic. I tried it for several months toward the end of my treatment plan. I can't really say if it helped or not. I wish I had discovered this product earlier on in my journey.

Special Note: Here's a quick Top Five Borrelia Busters I Wish I Had Tried:

1. The Buhner Protocol, including the herbs Andrographis and resveratrol
2. Acupuncture for Lyme fatigue and neurological symptoms
3. The Rife Machine, an eletromagnetic machine for killing off Lyme bacteria
4. More homeopathic protocols
5. A detox protocol *before* starting antibiotics to give my body and immune system an even better chance to respond to all the treatments that would follow

Top Five Lyme Whisperer Dietary Dos and Don'ts

August 5, 2014

1. **Gluten Freedom**. I do adhere to a gluten-free diet. I was already gluten free when I was diagnosed. I felt that that put me one step ahead in terms of controlling inflammation in my body, which can spiral out of control with Lyme. For a while, I practically lived on quinoa (a gluten-free grain) and butter, as it was simple and not upsetting to my stomach, while taking my antibiotics.

2. **Protein Power, Fabulous Fats**. I do center my diet on lean protein and healthy fats. I have nuts and protein shakes for breakfast; turkey slices, hard boiled eggs, and SunButter sunflower seed spread with rice cakes for snacks; chicken salad, avocados, or veggie burgers for lunch; turkey burgers, tofu, shrimp, fish, omelets, etc., for dinner. *The MD Factor Diet* by Caroline Cederquist, MD, provides great guidelines for optimal protein intake and snacking suggestions.

3. **Low Sugar.** I don't consume much sugar. I treat myself to gluten-free brownies every now and again, but that's it in terms of sweets. I watch labels very closely, even for sugars derived for brown rice syrup or agave syrup, which are sometimes thought of as "healthier alternatives." I try to avoid these as much as possible too. Mark Hyman, MD, has several best-selling books called *The Blood Sugar Solution*, *The Blood Sugar Solution Cookbook*, and *The Blood Sugar Solution 10-Day Detox* that I found to be incredibly helpful.

4. **Dairy Detoxes.** About twice a year, I don't do dairy. I undertake a dairy detox, at which time I go dairy-free for four to six weeks. I would love to be able to be completely dairy-free, but I simply have not been able to part ways with cheese, especially of the feta and gorgonzola kind! I would, however, not trade my vanilla unsweetened almond milk for anything. I add it daily to my smoothies, drink it with my dark chocolate every evening, or have a glass for comfort at any time.

5. **Dark Chocolate.** I do consume approximately 10 percent of my grocery expense each week in the form of dark chocolate. Particularly dark chocolate bars at 86 percent cacao, as well as dark chocolate–covered almonds. Dark chocolate–covered antibiotics would have solved some of my compliance issues. Rich in polyphenols, I envision that my daily servings of dark chocolate are protecting the cells in my body, especially my heart and blood vessels, which have not been immune to the effects of Lyme. I envision that the polyphenol ring structure in dark chocolate is choking Borrelia (see chapter 4's "An Interview with Professor Polyphenol" to see a polyphenol ring choking Borrelia). Dark chocolate also lifts my mood and spirits and is usually how I end my day. It's my nightly reward for being productive and motivated, and it makes me *very* happy regardless of how my day went.

Top Five Lyme Whisperer Exercise Escapes

August 8, 2014

1. **Walking**. At my sickest, I still made sure to get up, out, and walk. I had been a runner, so this was "slowing down" for me. I was lucky to be well enough to walk. I walked to keep strong and healthy mentally and physically. I walked spring, summer, fall, and winter. I walked as faithfully as I took my antibiotics. Walking, for me, was medicine. I still walk, though I prefer to run now that I can.

2. **Push-ups**. Nothing makes me feel like a weakling more than puny arms. My goal was always to feel and look strong and to be in fighting form against Borrelia at any given time. I was too tired and too time-pressed to do a resistance training program. Instead, I did and still do at least fifty push-ups (two sets of twenty-five) several days a week. For me, feeling powerful and invincible is directly correlated to how buff my arms are.

3. **Wii Dance**. I love movement, and making sure I never stopped moving was important to me. I was afraid that if I stopped, Borrelia would overtake me. I made sure my aerobic workouts weren't so strenuous that they were counterproductive. Wii's "Just Dance" was much fun and just the right tempo. I did it on days that I didn't go walking. I still catch myself singing the tunes of some of my favorite dances, "Rasputin," "Viva Las Vegas," "Iko Iko," "Proud Mary," "Monster Mash," and "Wake Me Up before You Go-Go." On my more ambitious days, I took on Wii tennis (and Wii tennis elbow)! I still occasionally break out the Wii dance for exercise during the winter months. I still dance when the mood strikes me.

4. **Running**. I started running again after two years of antibiotics and other therapies. I started easy, with 2–3 mile routes and then completed my first 5K. It was all uphill from there, literally and figuratively! Over the next two years, I ran over 1,300 miles over all sorts of terrain, running anywhere from 3–10 miles at a time. Today, I am still running, even though it does not seem to

get easier. Each and every run feels like I am just starting again for the first time with those tired heavy legs. But I push through anyways. The one thing that makes it easier is always getting the brightest and most colorful running sneakers I can find—who *wouldn't* find it fun to run with ASICS Gel Noosa?

5. **Tai Chi**. I had taken Tai Chi prior to being diagnosed. I found myself using a lot of the breathing techniques I had learned to fend off relentless panic attacks that consumed me during the thick of my illness. I also found the martial art–like movements comforting, peaceful, and empowering. I would recommend Tai Chi to anyone and everyone!

Top Five Lyme Whisperer Right-On Resources

August 18, 2014

1. **Tick-Borne Disease Alliance (TBDA) and Lyme Research Alliance (LRA).** In May of 2014, the TBDA and LRA announced the intent to merge, which would lead to the largest tick-borne disease organization in the country. Together, these united groups will be a force for fund-raising and research initiatives while being a powerful voice for advocacy and awareness. During the writing of this book, I often visited both *TBDAlliance.org* and LymeResearchAlliance.org as leading information sources. "Find a Medical Professional" is one of the features at the current TBDA website, providing access to Lyme-literate medical professionals.

2. ***Out of the Woods* by Katina Makris, CCH, CIH** In the first part of her book, certified classical homeopath and intuitive healer Katina reveals the unraveling and rebuilding of her life and soul while in the clutches of Lyme. Unbelievably, her story seems like a suspenseful romance and horror novel while being an unapologetically honest biography at the same time. In the second half, Katina's work is a great resource, covering signs and symptoms, laboratory testing, antibiotic therapy, acupuncture, classical homeopathy, naturopathic medicine, Rife technology, and emotional healing. It is by far one of the most enjoyable and all-encompassing books on the subject of Lyme that I have read.

3. **The Lyme Disease Association.** I found the LDA to be a great resource for detailed technical and scientific information. I discovered one of the most comprehensive documents I've seen on Lyme at *LymeDiseaseAssociation.org*. Go to "About Lyme," then "Controversy," then "Conflicts of Interest in Lyme Rprt" to see it for yourself! You can also search the "Dr. Referral System" for Lyme-literate professionals.

4. **ILADS.** ILADS is the International Lyme and Associated Diseases Society. It's a nonprofit dedicated to the appropriate diagnosis and treatment of Lyme and associated diseases. This

organization strongly supports physicians, scientists, researchers, and other health-care professionals. It boasts in-depth treatment protocols and treatment updates on its website ILADS.org as well as a "Physician Referral" feature for finding Lyme-literate doctors. Dr. Nathan Morris, MD, the author of the foreword for this book, belongs to this revolutionary society.

5. ***Why Can't I Get Better? Solving the Mystery of Lyme and Chronic Disease*** **by Richard I. Horowitz.** Dr. Horowitz's book has obviously had an impact on me. It inspired entries in my own book, including: "Hermione: The Heroine of Haphazard Lyme Hell," "The Polar Express: The Bell Still Rings Part 3," and "World War L" (chapters 8 and 9). While it is complicated and technical, it is the world encyclopedia for Lyme in my opinion. A must have.

Top Five Lyme Whisperer Awesome Affirmations

August 20, 2014

Affirmations are encouraging thoughts and intentions that plant seeds of hope, belief, and success in our minds. Affirmations help us to achieve what we want with the power of positive thinking. Affirmations are even more powerful with a sarcastic twist, says the Lyme Whisperer. Below are five affirmations I created just for my readers.

1. I will not let Borrelia keep me in bed all day. I will not hide behind my fleece sheets. I will get up. I will face the day. I will be productive, creative, and positive. If I want to return to my fleece sheets later, I will.

2. When I look at myself in the mirror, I will not see "someone with Lyme" first. Lyme will not define me. Instead, I will see someone defined by career goals, dreams, hobbies, clean eating, invigorating exercise, family time, friend time, rest time, and guilty television pleasures on Bravo.

3. I will fully commit to my treatments, and I will be 100 percent compliant most of the time without whining, even when I'm really, really, really just so tired of taking so many pills and it's so not fair I still won't complain unless someone takes the time to listen and then I'll hear myself complain out loud, which will make me realize how lucky and grateful I am for the treatments that I do have.

4. I will acknowledge the pain that Borrelia brings, both physical and mental, but I will inflict more pain on Borrelia than Borrelia inflicts on me.

5. I will beat Borrelia, one day at a time. And then, I will help others to do the same. Because as Stuart Smalley from Saturday Night Live said in his Daily Affirmations, "I'm good enough. I'm smart enough. And doggone it, people like me!"

You Know You Have Lyme When . . . your friends call you the Prude because you refrain from drinking too much or staying out too late. But you don't mind because you've worked so hard to maintain the delicate balance between feeling well and not feeling well that that third glass of wine or staying out past 10:00 PM just isn't worth it anymore.

Whispers of Hope

August 24, 2014

Borrelia, the first time I read anything by Katina I. Makris, certified classical homeopath and intuitive healer, was in August of 2012, in an article from the New England edition of *Wisdom of the Heavens, Earth, Body, Mind & Soul.*

Two years later, I would find out just how much wisdom and soul this openhearted woman had to share. The universe was pushing for her and my path to cross, Borrelia. We had several friends and acquaintances in common. In addition, I had reached out to her after learning about her Lyme Light radio program and new book, *Out of the Woods.* Over a Mediterranean dinner of grape leaves followed by fish and greens drizzled in olive oil, we sipped our cranberry soda waters at Giorgio's Restaurant, trading chapters from our Lyme disease journeys.

Nothing is random. I was meant to meet with Katina that night. The evening sky was illuminated with a beautiful full moon, and I felt illuminated from within from Katina's words of hope. I knew I would be able to share that hope with my readers. In Katina's book, I found a reservoir of that same hopeful healing advice she had shared over dinner that had resonated so deep. Surely, Borrelia, you were shaken by these powerful, invigorating thoughts as they reverberated through me.

How did Katina move away from the sickness and suffering? How did she truly get out of the woods? What hope can she offer us? There are so many powerful lessons from Katina's book, but I will focus on one message that I believe truly gets to the root of all hope. Katina, after much suffering, finally acknowledged and addressed the emotional trauma Lyme disease had caused her—the fear, posttraumatic stress, anger, and grief. She realized that she would never fully recover otherwise.

As a result, she took deliberate steps to heal the emotional scars. She surrounded herself with the right health team, including a devoted acupuncturist. She let go of a marriage stressed by her physical and mental downfall. She honored the power of healing places, such as her new home and favorite swimming hole. And she engaged in her creative passion of painting. In doing all this, she confronted and resolved the trauma head on so that she could free herself of it and move forward. I also confronted my trauma, by establishing a blog and launching a book as a creative, therapeutic outlet. These outlets allowed me to release the feelings and experiences that locked hope within me. I, as does Katina, feel that recognizing and unlocking the trauma frees the hope hiding inside. Hiding next to you, Borrelia.

Katina poignantly describes mentally stuffing her anger and negativity into a hot air balloon and pushing these feelings off into the horizon. Her heart, mind, and soul would not be scalded by these feelings for a day more, now that they soared to oblivion. I also remember the day I released my hot air balloon. It was the day I was diagnosed. From that day on, I let go of the anger and the agony over my medical situation and my experience with the medical system. I let it go because I knew those feelings would be sandbags holding me back from moving forward with my recovery, Borrelia. In the Lyme community, we need to release our hot air balloons whenever the gravity of negative thoughts weighs us down.

Having dealt with the negative, traumatic, and angry thoughts, Katina describes how her heart and mind became inviting and open to her intuition. She was finally able to honor her inner powers of perception and self-awareness in order to heal herself and eventually others. She trusted her innate sense for what was best for her body and listened to it carefully. She reacted quickly when she responded well or didn't respond well to her treatments or environment and adapted accordingly. She kept you on edge and fought hard, Borrelia. Eventually, her journey even took her on an unexpected career path that led to her becoming an intuitive healer while still battling Lyme. As Katina said in her book, "There is no one answer. As much as I want someone or something to tell me how to proceed with my life, to tell me if I'll ever really be healthy again, I realize that I must find my own way and honor my intuition." The power and direction of our own intuition gives hope to us all.

But there is even more hope in the fight against Lyme than the promise of our own intuition, Borrelia. Just ask Charles Balducci, cochairman of the Board for the Tick-Borne Disease Alliance, or TBDA. The TBDA is dedicated to raising awareness, promoting advocacy, and supporting initiatives to find a cure for all tick-borne diseases, not just Lyme. The TBDA recently announced a merger with the Lyme Research Alliance, creating a powerhouse for Lyme research and a unified voice for advocacy. Charles was kind enough to grant me an interview and touched on advances in diagnostics, legislation, research, education, and awareness campaigns.

He discussed the need for new diagnostics that would not only be available by prescription or over the counter but that would have an accuracy rate of at least 95 percent. In comparison, many of today's diagnostic tests for Lyme provide less than 50 percent accuracy. While the science that will deliver such a test is still being developed, the TBDA will work to further this effort. Ticktock, Borrelia. Can you *feel* the progress? Your days evading us are numbered like the face of a clock.

The TBDA also maintains a biobank. It recruits donors from all stages of Lyme and allows for blood samples to be "banked" for research purposes. Charles imagines the day when the new diagnostics will be used to screen samples from the biobank, providing the most accurate and comprehensive diagnostic database for Lyme ever.

We also discussed the TBDA's physician training program, a program in which health professionals are taught how to assess and treat Lyme. There is much hope for the growth of this program and others like it, which will improve access to physicians qualified to deal with this epidemic.

We optimistically discussed recent legislative efforts in states including New York, Vermont, New Hampshire, and Connecticut. These initiatives include Lyme task forces, Lyme Awareness Month, Lyme testing symposiums, bills that would protect physicians who prescribe long-term antibiotics, and bills that require insurance companies to offer coverage for long-term treatment. As Charles indicates, these types of state-by-state efforts will have ripple effects, as other states follow. These examples indeed provide hope for far-reaching, ripples. Ripples that can eventually lead to tidal waves of change. Can you swim, Borrelia?

Even if you can swim, you can't outrun the five hundred doctors from forty-two states that will gather at the Fifteenth Annual ILADS (International Lyme and Associated Diseases Society) meeting in Washington, DC. Leading Lyme experts, including Dr. Richard Horowitz, will lecture for four days, covering topics from recognizing and treating Borrelia, Bartonella, and Brucellosis to cutting-edge research and the latest in diagnostics from around the world. To imagine a ballroom at the Grand Hyatt hotel filled with an army of physicians determined to end the suffering is skin tinglingly hopeful.

Still, Charles believes, as does Dr. Nathan Morris as indicated in his foreword of this book, that the biggest waves will be made by the grassroots efforts of patient advocates. These advocates—who create Lyme organizations, protests, books, blogs, radio programs, bike tours, and more arc generating a forceful groundswell of awareness that will ultimately lead to action at the highest levels. Consider the example of John

Donnally, a twenty-four-year-old Lyme sufferer and cyclist who rode four thousand miles for the TBDA's Bite Back for a Cure cross-country bike tour campaign, raising awareness for Lyme as well as other tick-borne diseases. Having achieved this first challenge, John now has a goal of completing awareness bike rides in all fifty states, starting with New York, California, and Alabama. This level of awareness would not happen if not for the passion and self-directed efforts of John and others like him in the Lyme community. And everyone from the general public to legislators will take notice. They'll have to. Lyme advocates are too vocal and too active to ignore. It's up to me, you, and people like John. It is we who are at the heart of all hope.

I leave you, dear readers and Borrelia, with these parting thoughts, paraphrased from the words of Katina: These years spent battling Lyme have not been wasted. Where in the past we may have identified ourselves by our income, independence, and invincibility, we transform into resilient souls that identify ourselves instead with creativity, gratitude, and loving compassion. We grow and reflect in the hours spent in solitude, silence, and stillness. We gain perspective, depth, breadth, and balance in our lives. We find purpose in an unanticipated awakening.

These are the whispers of hope.

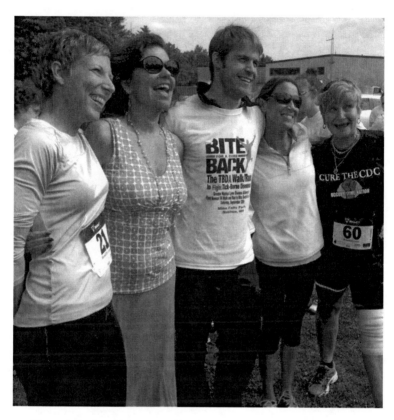

From left to right, Joy Pelletier Devins (Lyme Whisperer),
Katina Makris (author), John Donnally (of the TBDA),
Kelly Downing (of the Greater Nashua Lyme Alliance),
M. A. O'Connor (of the Greater Nashua Lyme Alliance)
at the first annual Bite Back for a Lyme Cure 5K run/
walk in which we raised over $10,000.

Index

CPSIA information can be obtained at www.ICGtesting.com
Printed in the USA
BVOW07s0051180215

388149BV00001B/67/P